W9-CMJ-169

August 15, 1997

with all best wishes
for a satisfying and
successful venture at
Bradley and Brown —

Tony Davids

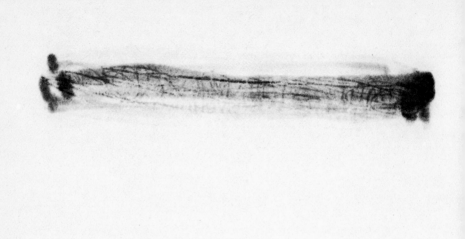

CHILD PERSONALITY AND PSYCHOPATHOLOGY: CURRENT TOPICS

CHILD PERSONALITY AND PSYCHOPATHOLOGY: CURRENT TOPICS

VOLUME 2

Edited by

ANTHONY DAVIDS, Ph.D.
Brown University

A WILEY-INTERSCIENCE PUBLICATION
JOHN WILEY & SONS, New York • London • Sydney • Toronto

Copyright © 1975 by John Wiley & Sons, Inc.

All rights reserved. Published simultaneously in Canada.

No part of this book may be reproduced by any means, nor transmitted, nor translated into a machine language without the written permission of the publisher.

Library of Congress Cataloging in Publication Data:

Davids

CHILD PERSONALITY AND PSYCHOPATHOLOGY: CURRENT TOPICS, VOL. II

74-7030

ISBN 0-471-19700-9

Printed in the United States of America

10 9 8 7 6 5 4 3 2 1

Contributors

Arthur M. Arkin, City College of the City University of New York

C. Keith Conners, Department of Psychiatry, University of Pittsburgh Medical School, Western Psychiatric Institute, Pittsburgh, Pennsylvania

Mary Engel, Department of Psychology, City College of the City University of New York

Norman Garmezy, Department of Psychology, University of Minnesota, Minneapolis, Minnesota and School of Medicine, University of Rochester, Rochester, New York

Robert M. Liebert, Department of Psychology, State University of New York at Stony Brook

Sarnoff A. Mednick, Graduate Faculty Center, New School for Social Research, New York, New York

Herbert Nechin, Department of Psychology, City College of the City University of New York

Rita Wicks Poulos, Department of Psychology, State University of New York at Stony Brook

Kenneth Purcell, Department of Psychology, University of Denver, Denver, Colorado

Fini Schulsinger, University of Copenhagen, Denmark

Hanne Schulsinger, Psychologisk Institut, Copenhagen, Denmark

Preface

The purpose of this series of edited volumes is to show the progress being made in the understanding of personality and psychopathology in children and youth. It presents topics of current interest to clinicians and theoreticians, and includes reports of work being conducted on the frontiers of psychological, educational, and psychiatric research. These books are designed as reference sources for researchers, educational reading for academicians and members of the helping professions, and texts for advanced students in courses on child psychology, personality, and abnormal psychology.

Each volume consists of original papers prepared especially for these purposes. Most of the papers are largely empirical, describing research projects and presenting findings from these projects. Other papers, however, present integrative reviews of relevant literature or critical evaluations of significant issues within this broad field. Over a period of years this series will publish papers devoted to most of the topical areas found in conventional text books on psychopathology of childhood. For example, among them are papers devoted to aspects of psychiatric diagnosis and classification, psychological assessment, learning disorders, hyperkinesis, delinquency, mental retardation, psychosomatic disorders, neuroses, and psychoses. The effectiveness of various forms of treatment are also considered, including residential treatment, special education, psychotherapy, family therapy, behavior therapy, and drug therapy. Naturally, such an extensive array of significant topics cannot be considered within the confines of any single volume. Some topics will appear repeatedly in succeeding volumes, but with new contributions prepared by different authors. Within any one volume, a given topic or issue may be covered by more than one contributor, but with different foci, methods, and/or findings.

The exact nature and contents of each volume depends on the timeliness and significance of topics and the progress currently being made by scholars and researchers. Many of the papers are highly controversial, and all of them focus on problems that are far from adequately resolved. These presentations are not designed primarily to settle issues or to provide only proven facts and final answers. Rather, they are intended to stimulate critical thinking, and to present a panoramic view of the wide terrain in great need of future creative thought and, even more important, much hard empirical work in the years ahead.

Whatever heuristic value and scholarly significance these volumes are found to have will depend essentially upon the calibre of the works submitted by the individual authors who accept my invitation to contribute papers. As editor of this series, I am indebted to these authors, all of whom are vigorous workers in varied academic and clinical settings.

ANTHONY DAVIDS

Providence, Rhode Island

Contents

CHILD PERSONALITY AND PSYCHOPATHOLOGY: CURRENT TOPICS

INTRODUCTION

This is the second volume in a planned series of publications focusing on personality development and psychopathology in children. It contains six original papers writen by leading authorities expressly for publication in this collaborative venture. These contributions are grouped into the following three categories: Part I, Cognitive and Personality Development; Part II, Psychophysiologic and Behavior Disorders; and Part III, Childhood Psychoses.

Part I opens with a paper by Engel, Nechin, and Arkin describing and presenting findings from a program of research on aspects of mothering related to cognitive development in first-born black male infants. This report integrates data collected from three vantage points—infant tests, home observations, and maternal interviews—over an eight-month period during the infants' second year of life. Naturalistic home observations in an urban ghetto are described in a vivid and moving presentation. For these researchers, the experience of making home visits to some of the most dreary living quarters in Harlem was obviously quite upsetting, and sometimes even frightening. However, even in uniformly dilapidated buildings, the researchers found a rather remarkable diversity of living quarters established by individual mothers, with some managing to establish pleasant and comfortable quarters where others had done nothing to make the inside of their rooms any better than the unattractive external surroundings.

In addition to these differences in physical settings, the researchers noted a variety of patterns of mothering among the women in this study. These differences are exemplified in a beautifully written segment of the report devoted to portraits of three women and their infant sons. Reading about some of the more troubled mothers and their troublesome infant sons, one can only expect that from such unhappy beginnings the path ahead for both mother and child is almost certain to be frustrating and unsatisfying. Other case vignettes, however, reveal mother–child interactions that are so full of love and mutual appreciation that one can at least hope that together they will somehow manage eventually to transcend the restrictive physical reality in which they now live.

The basic hypothesis investigated in the home observation phase of this study is that a significant portion of the variance on Bayley Scales of infant mental and motor functioning can be accounted for by maternal stimulation in the home. Actually, three clusters of maternal behavior are discussed: affective stimulation, nurturance, and encouragement of competence. It was found that at 14 months of age, sedentary stimulation in the home varies negatively with Bayley mental scores, while encouragement of competence varies positively with cognitive attainment. Engel and her colleagues state, "Where the mother behaves like a teacher, the baby is brighter, where the mother soothes and pets, the baby is less advanced cognitively, at 14 months of age." However, they caution against assuming causality here. They point out that brighter boys may *elicit* different maternal acts, and there may also be complex interactions in this regard that are not being measured in the present study. They alert the reader to be aware of this in viewing most of their reported results: one cannot be certain whether the mother's behavior is "causing" the child's behavior, or vice versa.

This investigation obtained quite different findings at 18 months of age than at slightly earlier or later ages. For example, only at 18 months of age did maternal reward and affective contacts correlate positively with results on the Bayley scales. According to the authors, their findings "lend support to Mahler's observation that there is a qualitative shift in the mother–child relationship at 18 months."

Turning to the maternal interviews, the following four major clusters of concepts were used in quantifying the content: maternal language, control, time sense, and psychological mindedness. Engel et al. attempt to answer such questions as: "Do aspects of maternal language explain variations in infant intelligence?" Interestingly, in this regard, the authors report that while these women generally were agreeable and cooperative, only a few were willing to take the Wechsler Adult Intelligence Scale. The investigators felt that this refusal stemmed primarily from the layman's hostility toward intelligence testing, and especially so in the case of testing minority group members. At any rate, they ceased trying to persuade the women to take the WAIS and instead substituted various linguistic analyses of the interview data. While not perfectly clearcut, with some variations at different age levels and when using different measures, the findings suggest that "the amount of talking on the part of the mother is significantly implicated in the infant's cognitive development in the second year of life."

Another question posed in this study asks, "Does psychological mindedness in mothers explain variations in infant intelligence?" As defined here, psychological mindedness consists of three continua: mother's affectionate response to the infant, her concept of developmental change, and behavior shaping. To measure this maternal characteristic, the women were presented with descriptions of ten critical incidents in which mothers often find themselves, each requiring some kind of evaluation, decision, and action on the mother's part. Some very interesting case illustrations of psychological mindedness are presented, along with statistical evidence of certain significant relations between this maternal attribute and infants' performance on the Bayley scales.

A general conclusion from this research is that different facets of maternal attitudes, feelings, and actions are relevant for the infant's cognitive development at different times in the period from 14 to 22 months of age. Based on their research to date, which is far from complete, the authors discuss possible implications for future social planning. They emphasize that not all babies being reared in the ghetto were faring poorly or needed outside intervention —some were doing perfectly well under their mother's care and guidance. But there were also some mothers " . . . whose life circumstances and whose relationships with their infants forecast nothing but catastrophy." As an innovative approach to prevention of such catastrophies, Engel and her co-authors suggest a Headstart program for prospective mothers during their adolescent years, *prior* to their having children. It seems highly possible that this form of cognitive preparation for motherhood would achieve much more beneficial results than attempts at working therapeutically with teenage mothers after they give birth to their children and are living in the throes of emotional turmoil.

In the second chapter, Liebert and Poulos report that by age 16 most children in the United States have spent more time watching television than going to school. Since, as they also report, television sets are now found in 98 percent of homes, almost all children have the daily opportunity to engage in this activity. The authors ask, "What, if any, are the socializing effects of this massive diet of television entertainment upon the young?" They then proceed to outline what is currently known about relations between TV viewing and personality development, emphasizing research conducted within the social learning tradition. Media influences are conceptualized in terms of observational learning, involving three major stages: exposure, acquisition, and acceptance. This framework is employed throughout the chapter to study the socializing effects of TV on child viewers.

Liebert and Poulos analyze the portrayal of aggression and violence on TV entertainment, and report that (1) aggressive acts are usually shown as the most successful way of reaching goals, and (2) the aggressor is most likely a white male. In exploring the impact of this TV violence, they review many experimental studies as well as correlational field studies. The evidence points quite conclusively to a significant effect of TV viewing on children's aggressive behavior. In this regard, it should be noted for interested readers that Volume 1 of the persent series (Davids, 1974) contains a detailed report of research conducted by Leonard Eron and his co-workers that represents the most comprehensive investigation of this topic to date. Findings from that 10-year longitudinal study, in which the same children were followed from age 9 to age 19, are cited in the present chapter by Liebert and Poulos as providing evidence of a causal link, rather than merely a correlation, between TV viewing and behavioral aggression.

Major segments of this chapter are devoted to discussion of roles and stereotypes assigned to members of various groups, including blacks, women, ethnic groups, and those from different occupational and social classes. Two basic concepts employed here are recognition and respect. Analyzing the content of TV programs in the earlier days of this entertainment medium in comparison with more recent programming reveals some very interesting indicators of changes in recognition and respect accorded to members of these various groups. Sex role stereotypes are given special attention, and it is obvious that a medium with the massive influence of TV could well have significant effects on changing attitudes toward behavior expected from boys and girls and men and women.

After reviewing and discussing the negative influence of TV through transmission of aggression, social stereotypes, and other troublesome behavior, Liebert and Poulos turn to "prosocial effects" of TV which until recently have been much less studied. The authors quote one authority who states that "All television is educational television"—programs intended strictly for entertainment actually do much to teach the young. Recent studies have been concerned with programs designed specifically to function as an educator of children, teaching them basic cognitive skills. Among these programs are *Seasame Street* and *The Electric Company,* which are produced by Children's Television Workshop, and have been shown to be remarkably effective teachers for children from both middle and lower social class backgrounds. Interestingly, to date relatively few studies have focused on TV's influence on interpersonal prosocial behavior. A study conducted by the authors of this chapter did show, however, that children's exposure to a prosocial *Lassie* episode led to an increase in their sharing and helping behavior.

A highly innovative development reported in this chapter is the recent attempt to create "television diets" to be used for purposes of research. Toward this end, a large number of TV programs were analyzed in terms of various behavior categories of traditional interest to investigators concerned with socialization, including altruism, sympathy, delay of gratification, resistance to temptation, and control of aggressive impulses. Through an elaborate system of analyzing and coding, ratings on these categories have been established for various TV programs and they can now be used for controlled studies.

The final segment of this chapter reports a collaborative research effort to develop 30-second presentations (termed "spots" and about the length of most TV commercials) designed to teach cooperative behavior through social learning. One spot, known as *The Swing,* depicts a potentially conflictful situation in which two children arrive at a cooperative resolution, taking turns using a swing and helping each other to enjoy it. This particular made-for-TV spot was first aired on network TV in May 1974 and has since appeared on all three major networks. Research reported by Liebert and Poulos has found viewing of this spot to be highly effective in promoting cooperation, rather than competition, between children.

In closing, it is emphasized that whether we study and understand it or not, this entertainment medium is having a major influence as a shaper of personality during children's formative years. This impact can either be ignored by behavioral scientists or made the focus of dedicated study; to Liebert and Poulos it is much too crucial to be ignored.

In Part II, we turn to psychosomatic disorders and behavior disorders. Here the focus is on abnormal personality development and psychopathology. In the first of the two chapters in this section, Kenneth Purcell presents an integrated summary of studies of psychological factors in childhood asthma. Relevant research by other investigators is cited, but the emphasis is on studies conducted by Purcell and his colleagues during the 1960s and early 1970s.

This program of research began with the observation that some children admitted to the Children's Asthma Research Institute and Hospital in Denver were "rapid remitters" (i.e., became symptom free shortly after admission, without medication), while others were "steroid dependents" (i.e., continued to show symptoms, and required drug treatment). Purcell asked the following question: "What are the factors which account for this dramatic difference in symptom response to institutionalization?" In the present chapter he describes the evolution of the research program aimed at discovering psychological determinants of differences between these two types of asthmatic children. Some of the determinants studied include parental attitudes and personality, family relationships, and child personality and emotions.

Purcell defines "asthma" and discusses hereditary factors that possibly play a role in the development of this disorder. He reports that the estimated incidence of asthma is from 2.5 to 5% of the population and, very interestingly, that about 60% of asthmatics are below 17 years of age. Moreover, this ailment occurs twice as frequently in boys, but the sex ratio evens out in adult years. In a recent collection of case studies of abnormal children, I noted "Another interesting observation is that this casebook contains more boys than girls . . . This finding is not limited to psychosis but is true for most types of childhood psychopathology, with a general incidence of about four to one in favor of boys. At the adult level, however, this ratio changes dramatically" (Davids, 1974, p. 222). I proceeded to speculate about possible causes and explanations for these empirical observations, and will not pursue them further at this point. But seeing Purcell's facts and figures pertaining to the incidence of childhood asthma makes me feel even more certain that sex differences in psychopathology at various developmental levels (including old age) deserve increased research attention.

In attempting to understand the variability found among asthmatics, Purcell describes three bases for subgroupings. One criterion is whether or not the symptoms remit upon admission to the hospital. Another is based on a measure of organic vulnerability to allergic symptoms. And the third is a psychological index derived from an interview seeking to measure the relative importance of different percipitants of asthma attacks as perceived by the child and/or the parents.

After providing this historical background and describing the types of procedures employed in his research, Purcell then describes an innovative and well-designed study involving experimental separation of asthmatic children from their families. Many interesting results from this research are presented, along with noteworthy attemps at providing meaningful interpretations of them. In general, the empirical evidence supported the conclusion that parental attitudes and/or techniques of managing the child's behavior are likely to influence the frequency of occurrence of emotional events that precipitate asthma.

The next major effort of these investigators was to gain more direct information about the role played by emotional states. They asked, "Is there a personality constellation or nuclear conflict specific to asthmatics?" They also decided that the best way to learn about functional relationships between emotional states and asthma attacks was to do so in naturalistic real-life situations. Purcell describes an ingenious procedure whereby a miniature radio transmitter was worn by the child, enabling the investigators to obtain an accurate simultaneous record of spontaneously occuring asthma and vocal behavior in the child's daily life. Findings from a fascinating series of studies are presented and discussed in this chapter; it appears that emotions of anger and excitement and the vocal behaviors of yelling and laughing were all capable of triggering asthmatic attacks. Purcell cautions that such findings were obtained in only some children, that the data are not yet completely analyzed, and that there is need for further refined studies to clarify some of the more perplexing results obtained to date.

The final sections of this chapter are devoted to discussion of the implications of the "subgroup hypothesis," both for clinical management of asthmatic children and for future research. In closing, Purcell presents two issues that he believes are especially important in the psychological study of asthma. One concerns the impact of the symptom on the child and his family, and the other concerns the impact that differing definitions of the problem have on the behavior of both researchers and clinicians. Purcell's observations and recommendations, based on extensive clinical experience as well as years of dedicated research, should be of value to all who are contemplating, or engaging in, work with children whose psychophysiologic disturbance can be so terrifying and even life threatening.

The second chapter in Part II is concerned with a topic that is one of the most controversial in the field of childhood psychopathology today (Davids, 1973). Under the title of "Minimal Brain Dysfunction and Psychopathology in Children," Keith Conners focuses on matters that are highly relevant to pediatricians and special educators as well as psychiatrists, psychologists, and parents. Minimal brain dysfunction is sometimes also considered under the heading "hyperkinesis," and these concepts are closely related to learning disabilities and problems in special education. This general area abounds with problems of definition, differential diagnosis, and treatment. While the perplexities of definition and diagnosis have been of primary concern to professionals who work in relevant fields, the use of drugs in controlling the behavior of hyperactive children has provoked great disagreement among both professionals and members of the general public.

In this chapter, Conners discusses the concept of minimal brain dysfunction (MBD), which he states is one of the most widely used, and most disputed, terms in the field of medical psychology of children. In attempting to understand this dispute, Conners traces the history of child psychiatry and the child guidance movement in this country, showing the early emphasis on psychological and environmental factors as having major influence on child development. Later studies showed associations between "organic" influences and disordered child behavior, including relations between pregnancy complications, childbirth abnormalities, and hyperactivity and disorganization in the offspring. In recent years, the term "minimal brain dysfunction" has replaced "brain damage," in recognition of the fact that although behavioral deficits are suggestive of brain involvement, definitive evidence of actual brain damage is rarely available.

Conners reviews some of the significant research showing the complexity of relationship between brain and behavior and cites studies in which expected relationships between organic impairment and hyperactivity were *not* found. Because of these contradictions, according to Conners, some investigators have come to view hyperkinesis as "a multidimensional disorder, with a variety of distinctive etiologies, only some of which are organic." Following his critical review of these various controversies, Conners discusses what he believes to be some powerful social and quasiscientific reasons why the concept of MBD has continued to have appeal and, in fact, to be used increasingly in work with children. For one thing, formulating these kinds of problem behaviors in children in terms of neurological impairment, rather than psychosocial disturbances, has had a heuristic effect by generating the search for new methods of treatment that might be more successful than the forms of psychological and educational therapies employed in the past.

Conners next turns his attention to the often-reported observation that hyperactivity may appear in some situations but not in others—for example, the child who is reported to behave perfectly acceptably at home but is described as a terror in school. He discusses some major differences that exist between home and school, and presents evidence from his studies showing the effects of situational stress on hyperkinetic children. This research has demonstrated quite clearly that when these children are asked to process information under conditions of distraction they fare very poorly. Conners draws upon information theory in designing these studies and accounts for the findings in terms of an interaction between "information load" and the hyperkinetic child's "distractibility."

The data obtained led Conners to conclude "that the pathology of a child may become apparent only under certain environmental conditions, and the role of treatments such as pharmacotherapy may depend upon the nature of the environmental demands placed upon the child." As he points out, these findings have profound implications for the question of under which circumstances medications might or might not be useful.

Another series of studies described by Conners examines the effects of stimulant drugs on the visual evoked response under three different conditions of stimulation (i.e., light, sound, or light and sound simultaneously). Some very interesting, but still not conclusive, results were obtained showing increased cortical activation under multiple sensory stimulation for some of the hyperkinetic children who were being treated with medication. Noting marked individual differences among hyperkinetic children, Conners proceeds to a detailed discussion of the heterogeniety found among children labeled as hyperkinetic or MBD. He shows that comparisons of global groups of hyperkinetics and normals often reveal no differences on the measures under investigation, while further refinements within the hyperkinetic category result in subgroups that do show noteworthy differences from normal control subjects.

Conners then describes fascinating recent research investigating the hypothesis that *some* hyperkinetic children are *under*aroused. Based on the findings obtained from measures of GSR and finger pulse volume, Conners concludes that when appropriately subdivided according to clinical characteristics, hyperkinetic children show lower autonomic arousal in response to repetitive stimulation and in situations calling for discriminations between competing signals than do normal children.

In the concluding segment of this chapter, Conners attends specifically to the topic of altering the central nervous system in hyperkinetic children. He discusses the use of amphetamines and related chemical compounds, but also describes several novel and interesting methods that are now available, including biofeedback, meditation, autogenic training, and other behavioral methods. Thus, while he maintains that psychoactive drugs have played an important role in developments to date, Conners sees newer methods of altering brain states becoming much more prominent in the coming decade.

Part III of this book is devoted to childhood psychoses, a broad and baffling topic that has become of increasing interest in recent years. Elsewhere I have discussed, and presented papers representative of, the continuing controversies concerning this most profound form of emotional and behavioral pathology in children (Davids, 1973). Moreover, Volume 1 of the present series contains three papers written by some of the world's leading authorities on etiology, diagnosis, and treatment of childhood psychoses (Davids, 1974).

The focus in the present volume is somewhat different, turning to another approach employed in attempting to understand the riddle of severe forms of psychopathology known variously as infantile autism, childhood schizophrenia, or childhood psychosis. This approach is often referred to as the study of "children at high risk," and usually is concerned specifically with children who seem more than likely to develop schizophrenia or other severe disorders. Some years ago, pioneering investigators decided that of all children, the ones at the highest level of risk for eventually becoming psychotic are those born to schizophrenic parents. As with other research concerned with normal and abnormal child development, the fathers are *not* included as subjects in most risk studies. Rather, the focus in most instances is on schizophrenic mothers and their offspring.

In the first chapter in this section of the present volume, Norman Garmezy presents a masterful coverage of the world's literature on studies of children at risk for schizophrenia, and also describes his own research program on "children vulnerable to psychopathology." In Garmezy's words, "This chapter provides a capsule description of some of the ongoing efforts to study the nature of vulnerability in children predisposed to the more severe forms of such disorders, and some of the central research issues involved in investigations of risk potential. The emphasis in this chapter is on predisposition to schizophrenia, but the restriction is an arbitrary one and the lesson to be derived from this seemingly narrow focus has broad applicability to the countless forms of behavioral deviance that plague mankind."

Garmezy perceives two foci of risk research: the study of *predispositions* (i.e., vulnerability) and the study of *stress* potentiators (i.e., life experiences). This formulation of deviance is sometimes referred to as the "diathesis-stress" theory, in which a vulnerable organism (resulting from biological, psychological, or sociological factors) is highly susceptible to malfunctioning in the face of stressful experiences encountered in everyday life. Interestingly, however, not all children who appear equally vulnerable are found to be equally unable to cope with stress, and these individual differences are of great concern to many who are now conducting "risk research."

At the beginning of his chapter, Garmezy discusses the current emphasis on children at risk, presenting some historical perspective and citing various developments that have played a significant role in bringing this research approach to its current level of prominence. A major factor was the growing disillusionment with retrospective approaches to the study of child development. Studies of normal children revealed considerable error in mothers' recall of their children's early experiences and past mother–child interactions. A closely related factor was the recognition that these interactions are not unidirectional, with mothers' behaviors influencing the children's development, but are actually interactive, with children's behavior also having significant effects on the mothers' fullfillment of their caretaking role. According to Garmezy, and other authorities whom he cites, to correct erroneous accounts of child development, retrospective studies must be replaced by ongoing longitudinal-developmental approaches in which the developing child, whether normal or vulnerable, becomes the center of inquiry.

In a major section of his chapter, headed "The Search for Children at Risk," Garmezy discusses the range of models that have been employed by various theorists and investigators to account for the etiology of psychopathology. Included here are the genetic model, ecological (or sociogenic) model, psychogenic model, and developmental model. For each of these models, Garmezy cites relevant empirical studies and points to the model's positive features as well as its limitations. According to Garmezy, "At this point in our science the choices among models are several and the need for a coexistence of diversity seems in order at least until the predictive power of each model can be resolved."

Having provided this historical and theoretical background, Garmezy then describes several illustrative programs of risk research. Here, in Table 2, Garmezy presents a tabular outline of "current programs of prospective research on children at risk for schizophrenia and related disorders." The comprehensive and detailed information provided in this table should provide an invaluable reference source for all students and professionals who become seriously interested in risk research. In my view, this table of information alone, which Garmezy gratefully acknowledges as being an expanded version of one provided recently by Erlenmeyer-Kimling, makes a sufficiently important contribution to warrant widespread utilization of the present chapter.

The later portions of Garmezy's chapter are devoted to detailed description and discussion of two programs of research into children's vulnerability to disorder: the Minnesota project and the Rochester project. Descriptions of aspects of these projects have appeared elsewhere over the years, and findings from specific studies within these projects have also been presented in various professional journals, book chapters, and unpublished reports. In the present chapter, we obtain an overview of these two major research programs, learn of some of the most interesting results obtained to date, and are informed of extensions of the research planned for the future.

The Minnesota studies include four separate groups of children at risk: one with schizophrenic mothers, a second with non psychotic disturbed mothers, a third group consisting of disordered children classified as "externalizers," and a fourth group consisting of "internalizers." Children in the third and fourth groups were being treated at child guidance clinics. Thus, for two of the groups the mothers are known to be psychiatrically disturbed, while for the other two groups it is the children who have demonstrated psychopathology. Garmezy describes the four-stage design of this research project, the general goals of which are (1) to describe and measure competence qualities in these children, and (2) to find response parameters that differentiate between adaptive and maladaptive children within the risk groups as well as between the risk and normal control samples. Several specific studies are described, showing the kinds of research being conducted at the various strategic stages in this long-range program.

In the closing comments of this chapter, Garmezy states, "Our current gropings reflect primitive first steps toward understanding the nature of vulnerability in these children. Hopefully, in time, a more sophisticated awareness of the qualities of the risk child will . . . provide us with methods that will help these children develop more effective ways of coping with adversity." When a dedicated, informed, and experienced investigator of Garmezy's stature, who is actively engaged in two of the major risk research programs in the country, refers to our present state of accomplishment as "primitive," we obviously have a tremendously long way to go.

In the final chapter of this volume, Mednick, Schulsinger, and Shulsinger describe and discuss one of the pioneering research projects on schizophrenia in offspring of schizophrenic mothers. In 1962 this "at-risk" research began studying a large sample of children of schizophrenic mothers in Copenhagen and has followed them throughout the intervening years. As Mednick and the Schulsingers state in the present report." . . . we have seen these individuals' lives follow a variety of courses; some have led rather 'successful' lives; some have succumbed to a variety of mental disorders; others have been repeatedly apprehended for criminal offenses." The most recent followup examination of these children was completed in late 1974, and included a thorough diagnostic interview. Here the authors describe the rationale and procedures of their high-risk method, present some findings from earlier stages of the research, and discuss the initial results stemming from the most recent diagnostic assessment. Also included here is a preliminary report of some premorbid characteristics of individuals in their study who have become schizophrenic.

Mednick and his colleagues review various approaches to the study of schizophrenia that have been employed most frequently in the past, and find them to possess serious limitations. They also state that "the long-term longitudinal study of children at high risk for schizophrenia is not without problems." Overall, however, they find several advantages in the high-risk design, and thus they turned from the study of schizophrenic patients to the prospective and longitudinal study of 207 young children with schizophrenic mothers, comparing them with 104 normal controls. They plan to follow their high risk and normal subjects for 20–25 years, and estimate that "During the course of these years . . . approximately 100 of the high-risk children will succumb to some form of mental illness, 25–30 should become schizophrenic."

At the start of the research program, pregnancy and childbirth records and early school reports were obtained, a comprehensive battery of psychophysiological, intellectual, and personality tests was administered, and psychiatric interviews were conducted with the parents and children. As of 1967, the first wave of 20 breakdowns in the high-risk group had been identified. Labeled the "sick group," these individuals were matched and compared with 20 high risk children who had not become "sick" but actually had shown improved adjustment in the course of these five years (the "well group"). In the present chapter, the authors describe the conditions characteristic of the sick group and compare them with the well group. Findings within the sick group are discussed in terms of autonomic functioning and possible neurological impairment, and are considered in relation to what Mednick has referred to as "a microtheory of schizophrenia."

In keeping with their research design, in 1972, when the average age of their subjects was 25 years, Mednick and his colleagues conducted another diagnostic assessment. This assessment included psychophysiological and cognitive tests, a social interview, and a battery of diagnostic devices. Included at this time were the *Current and Past Psychopathological Scales* (CAPPS) and *Present Status Examination* (PSE), both of which yield computer scored diagnoses. Clinical diagnoses were also formulated on the basis of the interviewer's evaluations, and very high reliability was established between the clinical and the CAPPS computer derived diagnoses. For purposes of the present report, the investigators utilized only the interviewer's diagnoses, and they emphasize the tentativeness of their preliminary findings. But with these cautions, they discuss some of the earlier life experiences found characteristic of those who at this time were diagnosed as schizophrenics. Implications of these findings for the early detection and possible prevention of severe psychopathology are discussed, and the authors state clearly that this is the primary contribution to be derived from high-risk studies.

They then proceed to illustrate this function of risk research by describing an intervention project currently underway on the island of Mauritius. Conducted by Mednick, Schulsinger, and a team of other investigators, "The purpose of the project is to select from the results of a population survey, three-year-old children at high risk for psychological disorder, place these high-risk children into therapeutic nursery schools, engage in specific controlled intervention and follow these children to observe their long-term outcome." Based on their previous findings of deviant autonomic functioning in the Copenhagen subjects who suffered psychiatric breakdown, and because of the probable cross-cultural stability of the measures, they used psychophysiological techniques to select the high-risk children in the Mauritian project. The present chapter contains a description of this research setting, the design of the study, and the various medical, physiological, and psychological examinations that were conducted with 1800 children between August 1972 and July 1973. Thus, this long-range prospective investigation is now in a relatively early stage. In the years ahead, we can eagerly look forward to what are certain to be valuable, and previously unavailable, findings relevant to the understanding and prevention of childhood psychopathology.

As indicated by the title of the present volume, the major purpose of this series of edited works is to provide students, clinicians, and researchers with the latest information about significant "current topics" in this broad field of child personality and psychopathology. The chapter by Mednick and his collaborators fullfills this purpose most admirably, closing with a description of their currently active and innovative research project, and leaving us to anticipate and speculate about the future yield.

REFERENCES

Davids, A. *Issues in abnormal child psychology.* Monterey, California: Brooks/Cole, 1973.

Davids, A. *Children in conflict: A casebook.* New York: Wiley, 1974.

Davids, A.(Ed.), *Child personality and psychopathology: Current topics.* Vol. 1. New York: Wiley-Interscience, 1974.

PART ONE

Cognitive and Personality Development

CHAPTER 1

Aspects of Mothering: Correlates of the Cognitive Development of Black Male Infants in the Second Year of Life*,†

MARY ENGEL, HERBERT NECHIN, and ARTHUR M. ARKIN

INTRODUCTION

The last twenty-five years have witnessed a remarkable upsurge of interest in the psychological development of the human infant. Under the powerful influence of psychoanalytic formulations, learning theory, and ethology, direct observations of as well as theorizing about the nature of infancy is giving rise to a rapidly expanding literature about the development of babies.

Research concerning the fate of specific responses such as head-turning or smiling proceeds alongside investigations of more complex processes such as attachment and stranger anxiety. Personal qualities of the biological mother or the primary caretaker, long regarded as major determinants of infant behavior, are also coming into sharper focus. Social awareness about the needs of "high-risk" infants and children brings with it increasing pressure for planning

*This research was supported by the National Institute of Mental Health (MH 17580-0351) and The Grant Foundation. Funds were administered by both the Department of Psychiatry, Montefiore Hospital, Albert Einstein College of Medicine and the City University of New York. Data were collected in the homes of subjects as well as at the Psychological Center, The City College of the City University of New York, 3332 Broadway, New York, N.Y. 10031. Principal investigators were: Wells Goodrich (now at the University of Rochester Medical School), and Mary Engel and William King, both at the City College of the City University of New York. The three principal investigators together with Herbert Nechin, the second author of this report, shared in the work required to design and implement this study.
†Arthur M. Arkin, the third author of this paper, acted as psychiatric consultant and performed independent evaluations of the mothers from a psychoanalytic point of view. This work is still in progress as are studies of time sense in mothers and follow up of 16 mother–son pairs.

early intervention programs. The wish to create such programs further under-
lines the need for research the results of which are usable in practical situations
(Joint Commission for Mental Health of Children, 1970).

It is clearly too soon to evaluate the long-range impact of hundreds of
publications per year concerning infancy. One may provisionally conclude that
cognitive development in general, and its relationship to environmental influences in particular, will continue to stay in the forefront of many investigations. Selected variables thought to relate to cognition such as performance on
developmental tests, response decrement, and early vocalizations are high on
the list of priorities. Maternal influence on intellectual processes is forever an
exciting area, representing challenging methodological problems. Varied as it
is, much of the current work may be organized around the role of many kinds
of *exogenous stimulation,* its quantity, timing, and source, for there is no topic
concerning infants that may be discussed without taking stimulation into
account (Ambrose, 1969).

A developmental view of the vast field of infancy research soon reveals that
neonatology in psychology is becoming a separate discipline. Following the
time immediately surrounding birth, the first three years of life represent
another area with visible divisions, bounded by studies of early learning on one
side (Lipsitt, 1970) and investigations of language acquisition on the other
(Brown, 1973).

Researchers coming to the field of infancy from a clinical background were
among the first to observe and record the reactions of babies to various kinds
of environments. Clinically oriented writers have long considered the second
year of life a particularly critical landmark for personality development. Bett-
leheim (1967) considers it one of three critical periods for an autistic *Anlage.*
Frustation of the will to act on one's own behalf at this time may lead to a
life of withdrawal, a severance of commerce with the outside world.

Mahler (1968) emphasizes that from the beginning of the fourth quarter of
the first year of life, powerful maturational forces press the infant to explore
wider segments of reality. The onset of the "practicing period" brings with it
a shift away from the mother and onto the ever more comprehensible external
world. While the practicing period manifests itself in many behavioral terms,
behavioral changes go hand in hand with an "intrapsychic separation individuation process": the child begins to function as a separate person but
needs to do so with confidence in the emotional availability of the mother. The
following quotes express succinctly the importance of various sub-phases during
the second year of life:

> The practicing period culminates around the middle of the second year in the freely
> walking toddler seeming to feel at the height of his mood of elation. He appears to be
> at the peak point of his belief in his own magic omnipotence, which is still to a
> considerable extent derived *from his sense of sharing in his mother's magic powers.*
> (Mahler, 1968, p. 20)

and:

In the next eighteen months this "ideal state of self" must become divested of its delusional increments. The second eighteen months of life are a period of vulnerability. It is the time when the child's self-esteem may suffer abrupt deflation . . . During the course of individuation, internalization has begun by true ego identification with the parents. (Mahler, 1968, p. 23)

Spitz (1957) has long considered the second year of life a critical landmark for personality development. Speaking of the meaning of the negativism of the "terrible two's" he suggests:

The volitional use of the ideational content of negation in the semantic "No" gesture is beyond doubt the most spectacular intellectual and semantic achievement in early childhood. It plays a large role in the child's relations with his environment. And more important, it is the manifest signal of the child's exercise of the function of judgment. It is probably the first conquest of the gestural or verbal symbol of an abstract concept. (Spitz, 1957, p. 99)

Spitz elaborates considerably on the long-range meanings of the new level of integration that is achieved at eighteen months; the "triumphant slogan" of the "I do not want this" period cannot be viewed as only a cognitive achievement since it is a message of a new relationship mode with the mother, and by implication, with the outside world. Without the "No" there is no "Yes"; affirmation and negation are both the results of relationship and cognitive ability.

To the extent that one takes these clinical observations seriously, it becomes impossible to think of cognitive development, or of early intervention programs designed to enhance it, in isolation from the relationship with the mother or the caretaking environment. The clinical realities demand that we select relevant aspects of mothers and mothering and of the environment in which mothering takes place, and ask what relationships there might be between how well a baby can perceive, move, remember, imitate, and vocalize and whether he is under or over stimulated. Relationships between baby variables and aspects of the mother and the world that contains them can then be regarded as islands of order, some of which may later delineate where cause and effect reside.

Where the mother or the environment of the dyad is depleted, low in stimulation, or erratic in this regard, studying cognition of infants in a natural rather than laboratory setting is especially indicated so that we not confuse the effects of "cultural deprivation" with deprivation of a more private sort, for which broad-spectrum intervention programs might be wholly ineffective.

With particular reference to "cultural deprivation," a 1969 report at the meeting of the American Association for the Advancement of Science spoke of the period between 15 and 22 months of age as perhaps critical for the origin of the cognitive lag that is often ascribed to lower class and/or black infants. Summarizing some data of his own as well as work by others, Schaefer stated that there is no evidence of social class- or race-related deficit on the Bayley Infant Scales before the age of 15 months. By 21 months of age, however, children from lower educational and cultural groups can be expected to show a deficit, unless participating in supplementary programs which provide various kinds of stimulation (Schaefer, 1969).

Such data are difficult to interpret. If the difference favoring white infants is there so early in life, does it earmark all poor children, all black shildren, all understimulated infants, or just some, or is there perhaps an interaction among such variables? The question also arises: can one plan social policy on the basis of developmental tests alone or does one need to interpret test scores in the broader context of naturalistic realities of life in an urban ghetto? At that time of the inception of the present study, descriptive knowledge of urban life of black and poor infants was badly needed, and various intervention programs were being considered for "culturally deprived" children.

The present study then arose out of curiosity about the vicissitudes of the second year of life among black infants, homogeneous with regard to variables that need to be controlled in a study of cognition and mother–infant relationship. It was hoped that a broad-spectrum descriptive approach would be informative about the realities of life in an urban ghetto setting. Rather than compare black and white infants, it was thought that a close look at variations *among* black infants would be more heuristically valuable, particularly if correlates of the level of cognitive development and its course over an eight-month period could be found in terms of aspects of mothering. It was thought that the question of the intellectual status of black infants versus white infants was still an open one and ought to be raised anew, but by comparing a homogeneous group of black infants to a representative standardization sample. The emphasis was on defining and measuring psychological variables rather than on "cultural deprivation." The attempt was to answer two major questions: (1) Do our subjects also deteriorate in their cognitive functioning by 22 months of age (2) Are there interpersonal and situational correlates of the fate of cognition in the second year of life?

This paper is an outgrowth of a short longitudinal study of first-born black male infants between the ages of 14 and 22 months. The study was carried out from three vantage points and by three groups of researchers. One group assessed the cognitive development of the infants at 14, 18, and 22 months of age. Another team conducted time-sampled home observations at these same points in time and recorded the frequency of certain mother-infant interactions. A third group of workers interviewed the mothers at the inception of the study (when all infants were 14 months old), using an extensive clinical interview of over 100 questions. Some required brief answers and others called for lengthy responses, all of which were tape recorded and subsequently transcribed.

Since the three groups of researchers did not exchange any information during data gathering, this tripartite design allowed for hypothesis testing not only *within* each data domain but also permitted the testing of hypotheses *between* domains. For example, and most importantly, not knowing the infants' test scores permitted those in charge of the study of maternal personality to make predictions about possible relationships.

The present paper reports results pertaining primarily to aspects of maternal personality as they relate to cognitive development in infants.*

The pilot phase

It required several weeks to develop our measures and to work out procedures by which prospective subjects would be contacted. During this time infant tests, home observations, and interview data were gathered on ten mother–infant pairs, N's varying with what measures were tried out with whom. The pilot data became very useful later, particularly in preparing methods of interview analysis, because it allowed us to check reliabilities of rating scales without using up data from subjects in the study proper for such a purpose.

Selection of Subjects

It is important to alert the reader that sample selection began with locating *infants,* not mothers. Nevertheless, some of the selection criteria did apply to the mothers. But, from the point of view of the home observation and maternal personality studies, the women whose homes were visited or who were interviewed became part of the sample because their infants satisfied certain criteria.

Birth records were searched in the Bureau of Records of the City of New York for names of infants, all of whom were black, male, first born, of native American parents. Prospective subjects had to have an Apgar rating of 8 or better, a birth weight of 5 pounds or more with no congenital disease at birth. The birth record had to show that there was no maternal disease or drug addiction at the time of pregnancy.

A pool of 145 subjects were thus identifed. Of these, 86 agreed to participate

*At the time of the writing of this report a follow up study is underway of 22 mothers who volunteered to be interviewed again. Their boys are being assessed for cognitive functioning in their sixth year of life.

and 20 refused. The rest were ill, or could not be found. Those who became subjects lived in health areas 03–38; 85.10 and 85.20. These areas cover the part of Manhattan generally known as Harlem, as far north as 181st Street, but also include deprived sections as far south as 77th Street west of Central Park. Infant mortality as well as tuberculosis have a high prevalence in these health areas. Of the 86 subjects who agreed to participate, 10 were designated as pilot subjects. Of the remainder, 51 mothers actually appeared for the first round of infant testing.*

Mothers were first contacted by letter, explaining the aims of the project, the fact that transportation to City College would be provided, information would be kept confidential, and that for each contact a subject fee of five dollars would be provided. The letter was followed by a home visit by a member of the project; none of the interviewers or testers made home visits, in order to preserve the independence of the three teams. The visitor scheduled the first of three home observations. Following the one at 14 months of age, the mother brought the baby for testing on two different occasions. The maternal interview was thus the fifth contact with members of the project; by this time mothers were fairly comfortable with us and spoke freely of their lives.

About one-third of the mothers were on welfare at the beginning of the study. Yet, their educational level varied from 8 years to 2 years of college. At the time of the interview, five mothers were attempting to obtain their high-school equivalency certificate. Ages ranged from 14 to 34 years, with a mean age of 20.

The caretaking patterns in this group were varied. Of 45 mothers who provided us with usable information about caretaking arrangements, 84% were primary caretakers of their sons. Table 1 provides a breakdown of the various patterns of care at the time of the inception of the study.

Information regarding caretaking was coded separately for days, evenings

---

*Within this report as well as in comparing this one with previous publications (King & Seeg-miller, 1973), the reader will have to tolerate fluctuations of sample size. Reported N's vary between 51 and 27.

In the study of cognitive development of the babies, 51 subjects received tests at 14 months of age. By 22 months of age the N dropped to 27.

In the home observation study N's vary from 49 to 32. There are many reasons for this. For example, if an appointment was not kept by the mother at 14, 18, or 22 months, the opportunity to reschedule the home observation either did not arise or, by the time it could be arranged the infant may have been too old for observation at either the 14, 18 or 22 months.

At the inception of the study 44 mothers gave us *complete* and *audible* interviews. Two additional interviews could be partially transcribed, thus raising the N for some maternal variables to 46. Three interviews could not be transcribed at all and two mothers withdrew from the project before they could be interviewed.

Naturally, when correlations are run between domains of data, further variations in N are due to data being present in one domain but not in the other.

Table 1.   Patterns of Caretaking Among 45 Mothers of First-Born Black Male Infants at 14 Months of Age

Patterns of Caretaking	N	Percent of Sample
Primary caretaking by mother:		
Mother only	29	64
Mother during day and week-ends, family member in the evenings	3	7
Mother during the day, sitter in the evenings or on week-ends	2	4
Mother during day and evenings, grandmother on week-ends	2	4
Mother during day, grandmother evenings and week-ends	2	4
Primary caretaking not by mother:		
Grandmother during day and evenings, mother on week-ends only	3	7
Grandmother, sitter, or other adult during the day, mother evenings and some week-ends	4	9

and week-ends. Where caretaking arrangements were changed prior to the time of the interview, the arrangement prevailing at the time of the interview was recorded. It might be noted in passing that the varieties of caretaking patterns took us by surprise. It would appear from Table 1 that the distinction of "monomatric" and "polymatric" (Caldwell et al., 1963) is not sufficient to assess the varieties of caretaking patterns. We shall return to this point later.

In any event, most of the mothers had worked at one time in their lives, but after the birth of their children almost half did not return to work. Nine did return to work, the rest were either married or lived with their families or with other relatives. Only two mothers were living alone with their infant sons. About one third of the sample was on welfare. We must report this in such a vague fashion because some who were on welfare at the time of the interview, a few weeks after were not. Also, "being on welfare" had varied meanings for these mothers. Some regarded it as a transitory circumstance, others were plaintive about it and had a hard time financially. Still others lived with as many as 7 to 18 family members (the average baby in this sample lived with eight adults including his mother), some of whom were also on welfare, and the standard of living could thus be considerably higher than for those living alone.

Twenty of the mothers were married, the rest were either separated, divorced or maintained other varieties of relationships with infant's father. In some instances mothers refused to answer questions about the infant's father. But the thirty who were willing to enter into such discussion revealed that the fathers ranged in age between 15 and 39 years, with half being under 25 years of age. The average father was a high school graduate; otherwise their educational level varied from three having finished ninth grade to four college graduates. Occupations were also widely varied: there were clerks, truck drivers, policemen, skilled tradesmen, and five fathers were professionals. Two young fathers were still attending high school. While only 18 fathers were reported to be living in the same household as the mother and child, most had regular contacts with their sons. Only six mothers actively prohibited this.*

We shall now report some results of the work of the three teams: infant testing, home observation and maternal interview.

THE COURSE OF COGNITIVE DEVELOPMENT OF THE INFANTS

Since the results of this part of the investigation have already been published (King & Seegmiller, 1973), a brief summary should suffice.

One white male and one white female examiner administered the Bayley Scales of Infant Development (Bayley, 1969) and the Uzgiris-Hunt Scales (Uzgiris-Hunt, 1969) to 51 infants at 14 months of age. Retesting was at 18 and 22 months of age, by which time the N decreased to 27. Administration was counterbalanced with regard to tests and examiners; no order effects of any kind were found.

King and Seegmiller (1973) show that the Bayley Mental Scales have considerable short-range predictive validity. For the longitudinal sample ($N = 27$) a correlation of .62 was found between 14 and 18 months of age; an r of .70 was found between 18 and 22 months of age. The correlation between 14 and 22 months was .57.

The patterns of change revealed surprising variety. Of nine possible types of pattern all but two were present. Increases of 25 points and decreases of 40 points were seen in some cases over the eight months! This magnitude of individual differences in a sample especially selected for its homogeneity is remarkable and requires explanation. Speculation about the correlates or rea-

---

*We are indebted to Professor Barbara Dohrenwend for advising against the use of any existing social class classification in this project. Welfare status is heavily weighted in any scheme for assigning social class membership. As the above description indicates, the variety of *actual* living standards is enormous among mothers on welfare; the pooling of meager resources elevates the quality of life while social isolation reduces the efficiency with which resources are used. Generally, welfare status obscures these as well as differences in educational level.

sons for such large changes in cognitive functioning have to come from a data domain other than that of the domain of mental test scores.

Of the 51 infants tested at 14 months, 27 stayed in the study, that is, were tested at 18 and 22 months of age. The mean on the longitudinal sample (N = 27) was significantly higher than Bayley's standardization sample at 14 months (mean = 106, standard deviation 9.2). By 18 and 22 months of age the mean dropped to that close to the standardization sample. The mean decrease was seven points. While the decrease is statistically significant (t = 4.7, df = 26, p < .01), these results require rejection of the hypothesis that the cognitive development of black infants decreases to a level below the national norm by 22 months of age.

The short-range correlations on the Bayley Psychomotor Scale were much lower than in the case of the Mental Scales: .17 between 14 and 18 months, .38 between 18 and 22 months, and .42 between 14 and 22 months. The means at all ages were consistently higher than that of the standardization sample; the initial mean of 111 (standard deviation 10.8) was evident both at 14 and 22 months of age, again causing rejection of the hypothesis that black infants are or become inferior to infants in general.

In discussing their results from the longitudinal as well as the cross-sectional point of view, taking into account intercorrelations among tests, King and Seegmiller suggest that there is an "18-month effect," which they deduce from the fact that long-range correlations were often higher than short-range ones. They also call attention to the difficulty of testing at 18 months of age. We shall return to this in discussing the implications of other findings.

MOTHER–INFANT INTERACTION: NATURALISTIC HOME OBSERVATIONS

The time-sampled home observation method used in this study originated at the National Institute of Mental Health, in 1964. Howard Moss and Paul Wender carried out a pilot study of 15 mothers and their 18-month-old sons. The Moss–Wender home observation scheme was then applied to 40 families studied by Howard Moss and Wells Goodrich in 1965. They found interobserver agreement to be .80 for two-thirds of their categories. During the pilot phase of the present study, the second author of this paper together with Wells Goodrich found that the scheme could be applied to mothers from a social class group lower than the Washington mothers were. In the present study, interobserver reliability ranged from 82% to 90% for various categories.

Method

Two observers were sent into each home when the baby was 14, 18, and 22 months old. The original plan was to send only one observer, but the neighborhoods held too many dangers for a person alone. A minimum of 2½ hours was required for each observation. Four home observers attempted to make six observations a week, but because of missed appointment, illness, or exhaustion of the mother (a number of mothers worked during the night), an average of three observations per week were accomplished.

Observers were trained to record the occurrence of eight categories of behaviors:

1. *Maternal Affective Stimulation:*   affective contact, passive-sedative stimulation, excitatory stimulation, holding (three kinds of body contact).
2. *Infant's Affective Behaviors:*   gross activity, vocalizes, approaches mother, shows pleasure, protests and fusses, cries and tantrums, mouths, self-stimulation.
3. *Maternal Control of Infant:*   instructs, distracts, prohibits, punishes.
4. *Infant's Response to Maternal or Environmental Influence:*   submits or nonsubmission, resists barrier, yields to barrier, environmental barrier (gets stuck), eats and drinks.
5. *Infant's Autonomous Social Behavior:*   physical distance from mother, scrutinizes observer, approaches observer.
6. *Maternal Nurturance:*   initiates nurturance, nurturant response (to eliciting infant), refuses nurturance, mother's availability.
7. *Mother's Encouragement of Competence:*   talks, entertains, encourages performance, rewards.
8. *Infant's Cognitive Competence:*   manipulative complexity, instrumental response, imitates mother, and seeks instrumental aid.

Two home observers were white males. One observer was a fair skinned Puerto Rican female, holding an M.A. in Education. The fourth observer was a black female, holding a teaching certificate. She was working for the Ph.D. in sociology at the time.

The two observers were standing side by side, each equipped with a clipboard, data recording sheets, and stop watch. During four 15-minute periods observers checked the occurrence of maternal and infant behaviors that fitted the categories above. The four observation periods were interrupted by rest periods for the observers.*

The Experience of Home Observing

Descriptions of rating scheme methods and quantified results omit many of the important aspects of the situation, especially personal reactions and impres-

*Those wishing to obtain a detailed definition of categories are encouraged to write to Herbert Nechin, Ph.D., The Psychology Department, City College of the City University of New York, New York, N.Y. 10031.

sions. Excerpts from observer notes may aid other researchers in planning similar work. They will also explain why observers had to go in pairs to apply a method which had, after all, sufficient inter-rater agreement to be administered by one worker at a time. Thus, H. Nechin wrote:

. . . armed with name and address we went. It was frightening walking through the streets of Harlem. Sometimes we were stared at, at other times we were approached by addicts or alcoholics asking for money. Clusters of young men stood around the corner; a living reminder of the high rate of unemployment here.

Many of the buildings are old, but some are well maintained against all odds. Mothers complained that addicts tear off mail boxes and steal light bulbs from the halls. Baby carriages or strollers have to be lugged upstairs; left in the hall they would be stolen.

Upon finding the correct address we were often stunned to see a building which looked as though it had been under air-raid attack; broken windows were covered with tin. There was the ever-present odor of garbage, animal or human feces and the damp odor of fallen plaster.

It was not unusual to have to step over a human being, "freaked out," lying in the vestibule. Mothers reported fear of opening their doors; some buildings contained empty apartments full of addicts, as in a "shooting gallery."

Such buildings often contained surprising oases of tastefully furnished, clean and cheerful apartments. Colorful decor, plants and decorative objects lent such homes a cozy, pleasant quality. Up stairs covered with graffitti, past urine stained elevators, past several security locks, . . . a mother with an infant son, books, records, toys,—not many but some,—furniture repaired . . . babies playing with cereal boxes, pots, utensils, grocery bags.

In contrast, there were cavernous, dark, meagerly furnished flats, and others that were cluttered beyond imagination. In some homes the only stimuli were rodents chased by children, or roaches that the babies played with. In others, the street noise, people fighting or loudly playing television sets or radios were the stimuli.

A few apartment's were totally unfit for human habitation and contained a mother heavily drugged or for some other reason unable to keep her head erect and her eyes open. An unbelievable variety!

Further description of the homes is as follows: number of rooms ranged from 1 to 9 with a mean of 4; 87% of the apartments had windows; in 59% of the homes the television set was kept on continuously and 75% of the mothers spent time watching it while home observers were present; number of toys ranged from 0 to 21 with a mean of 6.

Results

The reader will recall that the home observation scheme required noting the occurrence, or rating the extent, of mother and infant behaviors that fell into the eight categories (as listed above). Note that of these, four pertain primarily to what the infant and four mainly to what the mother does. Note also that each of the eight categories is comprised of a number of variables totalling 41 behaviors checked or rated.

While this report focuses on selected mother behaviors in relation to the cognitive development of their babies, it is important to demonstrate that the number of significant correlations between home observation variables and Bayley scores exceeded what might be expected by chance. At each age level 82 correlations were obtained between the 41 home observation variables and Bayley mental and motor scores. This computation with 14, 18, and 22 months data resulted in 246 correlations. At the .05 level of significance, 12 ought to be significant by chance. Table 2 shows that the number of significant correlations exceeds this.

Table 2. **Summary of Statistically Significant Correlations Between Mother and Infant Behaviors Observed in the Home and Bayley Mental and Motor Scale Scores at 14, 18, and 22 Months of Age**

Age at Observation and at Testing	Behavior	r Bayley Scales Mental	Motor
14 months (N=49)	Mother encourages performance, infant makes instrumental response.	$.32^a$	
	Mother distracts.	$-.30^a$	
	Mother provides sedentary stimulation.	$-.33^a$	
	Infant shows manipulative complexity.	$.31^a$	$.46^b$
	Infant has tantrum.	$-.35^a$	
	Infant attacks mother.		$.32^b$
18 months (N=34)	Infant expresses pleasure.	$.34^a$	
	Infant imitates mother.	$.45^b$	
	Mother unavailable.	$-.49^c$	
	Mother rewards.		$.39^a$
	Mother punishes.		$.49^c$
	Mother provides affectionate contact.		$.59^c$
22 months (N=32)	Infant self-stimulates.	$-.37^a$	$-.39^a$
	Infant resists environmental barrier.	$-.39^a$	
	Mother talks.	$.38^a$	
	Mother instructs and infant yields.	$.34^a$	
	Infant imitates mother.	$.38^a$	
	Infant scrutinizes observer.	$-.43^b$	
	Infant yields to environmental barrier.		$-.38^a$
	Mother prohibits and infant yields.		$-.40^b$
	Mother holds infant.		$.39^a$

^{a} $p < .05$, two tailed.
^{b} $p < .02$, two tailed.
^{c} $p < .01$, two tailed.

The main hypothesis of the home observation study was that a significant part of the variance of the Bayley Scales at any one point in time will be accounted for by maternal stimulation in the home. The present paper is addressed only to data pertaining to this hypothesis (other aspects of the home observation results will be published at a future date).

The kinds of maternal behaviors most relevant to our hypothesis are: *maternal affective stimulation, maternal nurturance, and mother's encouragement of competence.* Table 3 summarizes the results. It is evident that at 14 months, sedentary stimulation in the home varies negatively with Bayley Mental scores while encouragement of competence (with instrumental response on the part of the infant) varies positively with cognitive attainment. These two correlations may mean that passivity-inducing stimulation on the part of the mother (stroking, petting, fingering, quiet talk) is not a suitable stimulus for cognitive development, at least not for first-born males, while interactions that require or elicit performance *and* succeed in obtaining it, do covary with achievement on the Bayley Scales. Where the mother behaves like a teacher, the baby is brighter; where the mother soothes and pets, the baby is less advanced cognitively, at 14 months of age. It is important to be wary of causal interpretation, for it could easily be that congenitally brighter boys *elicit* different maternal acts, and it may also be that there is an interaction too complex to tap by our methods. This caveat applies to all the results here, and will not be reiterated.

At 18 months, *affectionate contact* with the baby assumes a positive relationship to motor development, and it is interesting that only at 18 months does kissing, hugging, or nuzzling explain any of the variance on the Bayley Scales, and that it is *motor* not cognitive achievement that is at issue. Together with the significant correlation of motor scores with *mother rewards,* and the negative one with unavailability, this may mean that the motor development of the 18 month old is more at issue in the mother–child interaction and that affective aspects of interaction are becoming more relevant for motor and mental development than they were at 14 months. Note that *reward* and *affectionate contact* bear a positive relationship to Bayley scores only at 18 months. By 22 months rewarding relates negatively to motor skill. This may mean that 18-month-old boys are more able to elicit overt signs of love than they were earlier or will be later, during the second year of life. Or it may mean that mothers are more loving in their behavior when the infants are at the zenith of their celebration, sharing in the mother's power. Either way, this finding, together with the significantly negative relationship between cognitive achievement and maternal preoccupation with matters other than the infant, lends support to Mahler's observation that there is a qualitative shift in the mother–child relationship at 18 months.

One might say that by 22 months the importance of affective contact for mental and motor development continues; the correlations suggest that *holding* and *talking* have a greater role than before. The behaviors categorized under

Table 3.   Correlations Between Bayley Mental and Motor Scale Scores and Frequency of Various Maternal Behaviors in the Home at 14, 18, and 22 Months of Age

Maternal Behaviors	Bayley Mental Scale			Bayley Motor Scale		
	14 mo $n=49$	18 mo $n=34$	22 mo $n=32$	14 mo $n=49$	18 mo $n=34$	22 mo $n=32$
Affective stimulation						
Provides affectionate contact	−.04	.03	.13	.00	.59 [b]	.14
Provides sedentary stimulation	−.33 [b]	−.15	.18	−.21	.15	.07
Provides excitatory stimulation	.16	.21	.00	.14	.17	−.00
Holds infant	−.01	.07	.27	.00	.04	.39 [b]
Maternal nurturance						
Initiates nurturance	.01	.04	.06	.08	.13	−.02
Nurturant response to eliciting infant	−.01	.07	−.02	.20	.05	−.12
Refuses nurturance	−.01	−.10	−.08	.24	−.02	−.17
Mother's availability						
Totally free	.04	.15	.05	−.09	.05	.06
Socializes with others	−.16	−.19	.12	−.00	.08	−.17
Busy with work	.02	−.49 [b]	−.01	.12	−.10	.24
Busy with self-care	−.08	−.12	−.04	−.11	.04	.00
Cannot be observed	.08	.21	−.21	−.03	−.08	−.10
Encouragment of competence						
Talks to infant	.21	.12	.38 [b]	.12	.26	.18
Entertains	.15	−.12	.26	.04	−.07	−.17
Encourages performance, no response from infant	.13	.30	.11	−.01	.21	.12
Encourages performance, infant makes instrumental response	.32 [a]	.28	.32 [a]	.06	.17	−.27
Rewards	.21	.25	.17	−.16	.39 [a]	−.30 [a]

[a] $p < .10$, two tailed.
[b] $p < .05$, two tailed.

holding and *affective contact* involve touching, all the way from nuzzling and kissing to holding the infant's hand.

It is important to note that *nurturance, availability,* and providing *entertainment* do not explain any of the variance of either cognitive or motor achievement. How can this be? These categories include routine caretaking behavior, feeding, dressing, just being present, singing, or saying simple things like "look at the toy." The lack of relationship here in light of the positive relationships with definite affective behaviors suggest that, after 14 months of age, *maternal acts that are both structured and affectionate* may carry more weight than loosely structured behaviors; benign availability is simply irrelevant to cognitive development in the second year of life.

Maternal talk, double scored in the scheme, will be discussed in the following section of this report, where maternal talkativeness and the quality of language will be considered more generally.

MATERNAL PERSONALITY: INTERVIEWS IN DEPTH*

The purpose of the maternal personality study was to obtain an independent view of the mother, this time not in her home with her baby, but seated with another woman, discussing him for an hour or two, in a relaxed atmosphere.

The interview consisted of about 100 open-ended questions, some requiring brief responses, others calling for more elaboration. Since many mothers became quite engrossed with the interviewer, the latter followed the mother's train of thought, allowing rambling and sidetracking. This makes for a very good relationship.

The interview covered the baby's developmental history as well as present caretaking practices. The baby's habits, mode of relating to the mothers and other important adults, and to other babies was covered. The mother was encouraged to imagine the child's future, both in terms of practical matters like jobs and educational attainment, as well as in terms of the kind of person he is likely to become and why. Much of the focus, however, was on the mother. We were interested in her past, her childhood recollections, her experiences with caretaking before she became a mother. We explored major discontinuities in her life, such as moving North, deciding to continue in or to drop out of school. We asked about the people who are her major source of security and support, and about her worries and fears. We elicited a great deal of data about

---

*The reader will recall that mothers were interviewed at the outset of the study, that is, when their sons were 14 months old, that 44 mothers gave us complete and clearly audible interviews, and parts of an additional two interviews were usable. Attrition did not affect us in this part of the study, except when relating maternal variables deduced from the interview with home observations or mental test scores of infants.

her manner of using time, both in terms of a typical day and larger units of time. We ended the interview with a series of critical incidents relevant to mothers of children in the second year of life, inquiring how she might cope in these situations and why.

The interviews, tape-recorded and transcribed, yielded data ranging from 33 to 120 typed pages. They reveal a variety of personalities, personal histories, attitudes toward motherhood and life in general that boggles the imagination and challenges one's ingenuity in devising methods of quantification. Before describing the methods of analysis and results—only some of which can be reported here—the reader will gain a sense of the kinds of people the mothers were, through a few impressionistic descriptions, which albeit lacking precision of disciplined "description of the sample," may aid in increasing the reader's familiarity with the women we spoke with.

Portraits of Three Mothers

Portrait 1

She is in her early twenties and was married a couple of years before her baby boy was born. She and her husband live with the maternal grandmother in a small central Harlem apartment. She dislikes the noise, the dirt, and the addicts and has fantasies of moving out of the city. But her husband has all his friends there and he is linked in many emotional ways to where they now live. She has retreated from this conflict with him.

When she was pregnant she worked as a filing clerk and was learning key punching. She gave this up when the baby was born. The delivery was all right but problems began as soon as they were home from the hospital. He "didn't act right" and the doctor thought he "had a bad cold." Then things went well for a while until he really became ill and had to be taken back to the hospital. The diagnosis was asthma. It was frightening. It was as if he couldn't breathe at all. She thought he might die if she did the wrong thing. All this was in the second half of the first year of life. He is now 14 months old. He is such a problem that she wonders how she will manage at all. She certainly is not going to have any more children. He spits up when she feeds him; only the grandmother can manage smoothly with him. He will not sleep at night. He awakens constantly, wants things, awakens *her*. Then when she does want to play with him, he is sleepy and uninterested. He will not let her out of his sight. He screams and screams and works himself up to where she is afraid he might have another asthma attack.

Shortly after he was a year old the grandmother advised her to go back to work before she became a complete wreck and offered to take care of the baby.

She went back to key punching. She has to get up very early in the morning and she comes home around three in the afternoon. Now the matter of sleeping schedules is thoroughly confused. The grandmother lets the baby sleep until eleven in the morning to *make up* for some of the sleeplessness of his nights. He is then fed and bathed and is very lively. When she, the mother, comes home at three, she is tired and would like to nap, but he demands attention. From then on, until she finally gets him into bed, it is an unsynchronized battle, with almost no pleasure for her. Her attempts to escape to the neighbors do not succeed; in fact, she can hardly even go to take the garbage to the chute. He insists on coming with her to the end of the hall. She trots out, garbage in one arm, baby in the other. He is heavy, he fidgets. The garbage is thrown out, the baby clings or screams. How will he ever learn night from day? How will she ever get any rest? And what if he gets sick again? And what if none of it will ever work out?

What will he be when he grows up—or should she try to imagine? He will be a sly, mean man, because already he is a sly, mean baby. The grandmother says it is "bad blood"—he got it from an uncle who was bad like him. It must indeed be in his blood.

She is very thin, very tired looking. She moves quickly and sits prettily. She is not what one might call beautiful but she has good style and is very chic. She sits forward in her chair and smokes, and her eyes dart from objects in the room to tape recorder in a quick, alert way. Her speech is like that too, quick and tense. She leaves as she came, matter-of-factly, having cooperated, finding it all interesting, not asking for anything.

Portrait 2

She is barely out of high school and she is not married. She lives with her father, stepmother, baby, and the baby's father (also a teenager) in a crowded central Harlem apartment. Her parents were divorced when she was young and she did a lot of caretaking as a child. The children stayed with the mother in the South. She has only recently become reacquainted with her father, since remarried. She gets along well with her stepmother, who has no children, but continues to be somewhat ill at ease around her father.

She became pregnant in high school but wanted to finish. She giggles as she tells how no one knew she was expecting when she got her diploma. Although she was quite advanced in her pregnancy, this was possible because she is and always has been really fat. She stops short of being obese, but she is a big girl, with large breasts, heavy thighs and a fat, round smiling face. She is very comfortable with herself, has no intention of dieting, and moves, sits and carries herself in the manner of an older woman who is used to being fat and likes it.

The baby is nothing short of God's gift to the world. She could hardly wait to have him. She and her young man went shopping for the baby quite often. He usually darted out of the store in some kind of embarrassment, like when he asked a saleslady which part of the baby the bootees were for! He was laughed at and fled the store!

The young man is finishing some training course that she cannot specify, then they are going to get a place of their own. The family feels they shouldn't marry until he can support them, and this is fine with her. She wears an ambiguous-looking ring but calls herself "Miss."

Her main complaint is lack of privacy. Otherwise life is rather marvelous, what with the baby taking up her time completely and being such a fine fellow. He says words! He eats adult food! He began to drink from the cup all on his own! He tries to learn like when he walked up to her, looked into her face, and said very seriously, "Nice baby." As she tells this, she beams. Her eyes sparkle. If only she could think of more things to tell me! She imitates him and enacts how she talks to him and how he reacts. When he pesters her and she is doing her housework, she shoos him off. At such times he often has a tantrum. She won't have that. She spanks his legs. She talks seriously to him. He quits crying. She orders him into *his* rocking chair where he then begins to rock at breakneck speed, casting furtive, sidelong glances at her. He pouts. Finally she "forgives" him with a big show of love, gathers the baby to her large body, and bestows upon him a cookie.

She talks so much. I hardly need to ask questions, just enough to steer her around the ones I have in mind. The interview goes on and on. They lock the office, the janitor wants to leave. I ask her to come back another time to finish the other questions. She is delighted. She returns with a girlfriend, hardly older than herself, and we continue. Her supply of anecdotes is endless, she has a sense for the comic, a lusty, joyful attitude toward life.

Portrait 3

She was still a minor when she delivered the baby. She had to drop out of school and had to confess to her mother who practically skinned her alive. During her pregnancy she was tearful, lonesome, dejected. She had felt that way before because as a child she had a serious allergy and had to go to the clinic a lot. This was in the South. She recalls looking at older girls in the clinic who were wearing lipstick, thinking to herself that she would probably always be barred from fun because of her illness.

She really dislikes her mother, with whom she still lives. But she has a better relationship with her kid sister. She takes me up on the option to skip certain questions if they seem too personal, and so avoids talking about her father. But she will talk about the baby's father, whom she dislikes. He is no good, he cannot be counted on, and he will be a bad influence on the child. So, although she does allow him to visit the baby, she *decided not to marry him.* Occasionally she gives him some money. He is always broke.

She is a pretty woman with a collegiate look, courteous and considerate toward me and my machinery. There is an inner dignity, a kind of reserve; she is very likeable. As she tells about the loneliness of her maternity, tears come. Her mother wouldn't allow her to keep the baby. As a minor she was helpless. The baby was born and they sent him *to a foster home.* She begged and fought. She testified to her own worth. She finally convinced "them" that she could have custody of the baby if she demonstrated that she could provide support. She got a job working nights in a post office. It was bad, but she had to do it. She was not supposed to visit her son, but the foster mother was amenable and so she was able to see him about every two weeks. This was a secret from the grandmother who kept fairly close tabs on her. By the time the baby was six months old, she had shown that she could work and earn. She also obtained a high school equivalency certificate. She was awarded her son after she was able to obtain a daytime job. She now does filing for one of the major newspapers and is truly grateful for the good treatment she gets there.

She fights back her tears as she talks about her need for money. She cannot stay long with her mother and sister. She has already arranged for a sitter; she takes the baby in the morning and her sister picks him up in the afternoon. The sitter is expensive. Every penny she earns is spent on fares, food, the baby's needs, and the sitter. The subject fee she will get from me for the interview is needed badly, too, although she courteously tries to reassure me that the study is "interesting and worthwhile" in itself.

Yes, she has begun to go out. There is a new young man. Some joy in her face when she says this, but nothing like the feelings when she talks about her son. His rate of development, his quick use of words, his ways of anticipating happenings, his charm and his talents are then described with full details, showing that she is very conscious of the value of his achievements and planfully works at teaching him skills as well as language.

The Strategy of the Analysis of Maternal Interviews

From a formal point of view, interviews were subjected to four levels of analysis. These levels differ with regard to the mental operations necessary to translate interview data into numerical form. On the lower levels of analysis, concepts, theory, and inference played at best a minimal role. At the highest level of analysis, theory played a major role; what the mothers said was reformulated into sophisticated clinical interpretations regarding their motivation on various levels of awareness.

More precisely, interview analyses on Levels I and II required us to *count* and *code* those kinds of data that do not require judgment. The mother's age, the number of siblings she had, the number of years of school attendance—these kinds of information are given in quantities. Whether the mother plans to go back to work or not, whether she is married or not—these kinds of data can easily be coded.

Beyond that which can be counted or coded are vast riches of data that can be quantified only according to a theoretical orientation expressive of the investigator's choice of personality theory. The present study bears the obvious imprint of psychoanalytic theory; those concepts that were evolved to generate clinical judgment were chosen because psychoanalytic personality and developmental theory implies or assumes them to be important.

Here Level III analysis of interview data refers to the application of *clinical judgment* by experienced clinicians who have worked with mothers and children for five or more years, and whose clinical work is psychoanalytically oriented. These judges were chosen very carefully and were paid on a per-hour basis (an average of $25 per hour) to compensate for time spent in checking reliabilities of ratings or in performing ratings once the data started to accumulate.*

The level of clinical judgment necessitated dismembering the interview in order to limit halo effects. Generally, judges were asked to make a limited number of judgments, and variables were so assigned to judges as to avoid combining judgments of related variables. In seeking quantification of certain variables, interviews were offered to judges in parts, for example, where knowing the mother's own childhood history would have influenced judgment of the quality of mothering she was capable of, such information was detached.

Dismembering the interviews and offering them for judgment in parts was thus necessary for the sake of method. Yet, ultimately there had to be a time when each interview, each mother who spoke to us was viewed in toto, not as scoring high or low on this scale or that, but as a fully functioning person, comprehensible only in *all* that she said. This conviction led to the definition of Level IV, the total *pyschoanalytic interpretation* of each interview by a psychoanalytically trained psychiatrist who had ample experience in psychotherapy with black men and women. (This part of the interview analysis is mentioned here only to complete the description of the entire strategy composed of Levels I, II, III, and IV, representing counting, coding, clinical

---

*The level of expertise required to perform clinical judgments of interview data is a most important variable; the most elegant concept and most carefully collected and transcribed interview data may be rendered worthless by careless, uninformed, or contaminated judgments or by inexperienced raters. Number of years of experience combined with a relative homogeneity of theoretical orientation is the best index to confident judgments in general and respectable interjudge reliabilities in particular.

judgment, and psychoanalytic interpretation, respectively.) So much for the formal aspect of the quantification, that is, *how* quantification was achieved.

With regard to content of analysis, that is, *what* was quantified, we worked with four major clusters of concepts, under the headings of *maternal language, maternal control, maternal time sense,* and *psychological mindedness.* These concepts as well as the variables that comprise each were chosen before the onset of the study because they were seen as pivotal and minimally sufficient in understanding varieties of caretaking *and* because it appeared *possible* to obtain data relevant to these concepts from interviews. (That is, there may be other aspects of caretaking that would be very important to study relative to the cognitive development of infants, but not all may be illuminated by interviewing mothers.)

Of these clusters of concepts the analysis of maternal language required coding and very little judgment. Quality of maternal control did, however, involve the use of sophisticated clinical judgments to quantify the mother's tolerance for impulse expression, her sense of adequacy or helplessness when the infant was in a rage, the overall effectiveness of her methods of control, and the rigidity or flexibility in the use of various methods of control, all in relation to the infant's cognitive development (Wieder, 1972).

Time sense of mothers is currently under analysis and involves variables such as optimism, pessimism, and past, present or future centeredness in relation to various aspects of the mothers' lives as well as in relation to cognitive development.

Psychological mindedness is a three-pronged concept that will be defined operationally below. It attempts to assess the degree to which mothers' interviews vary in tenderness, empathy in teaching and shaping behavior, and the understanding of the reasons for infant behavior in terms of developmental level. Here we attempted to differentiate the extent to which mothers conceived of their infants as *psychological* versus *physical* realities. We attempted to capture the full range from delicate appreciation of malleability of an evolving human being to cruder perceptions of the infant as a little animal who needs to be housebroken and controlled.

Of the above listed clusters of variables in the maternal personality study, this report is limited to results pertaining to maternal language and psychological mindedness.

Do Aspects of Maternal Language Explain Variations in Infant Intelligence?

Previous research indicates that correlations between intelligence test scores of mothers and young children tend to be higher for girls than for boys and that they seldom explain much variance among children. Olim (1970) correlated the Verbal Intelligence Scores (WAIS) of 163 black mothers and their four-year-old children, using subjects from various social classes, and found a correlation of .30 between maternal Verbal WAIS scores and Binet scores. This correlation, albeit significant beyond the .001 level, held only for girls; for boys it was only .15. Olim interpreted these findings as corroborating those of Kagan and Moss (1959).

Such data, while of interest to the present study, were really not sufficient to reassure us that whatever relationships may be found between aspects of mothering and infant cognitive development might be due only to brighter mothers having brighter babies. This sample was younger than in other studies, and it consisted entirely of first-born males, none of whom had Apgar scores of less than eight. The select nature of the sample, and its homogeneity with regard to variables critical to intelligence, necessitated our own test of the possibility that maternal intelligence may explain much of the variance among the infants.

While generally agreeable and cooperative, only few of the mothers consented to take the Wechsler Adult Intelligence Scale. Their reticence could be explained by much laymen's discussion and hostile feelings against intelligence tests in general, and the use of tests with minority group citizens in particular. Incomplete intelligence test data on the mothers thus forced us to consider a linguistic analysis of their interviews; richness and structure of language is often a very close approximation to intelligence test achievement. We substituted various linguistic analyses and ceased trying to persuade mothers to take the WAIS.

The linguistic analyses were applied to 43 of the 51 interviews; because of limitation of funding we excluded interviews where much of the infant data were missing or where technical difficulties impeded accurate transcription.

The method of linguistic analysis may be summarized briefly. Since interviews varied greatly in length, that of the shortest interview, 33 pages, was taken as the limit for analysis. Beginning with the third page, every subsequent third page was analyzed.

To obtain a measure of the richness of vocabulary, each noun, verb, and modifier initially used by the subject was recorded on an index card. The cards were alphabetically arranged. Each subsequently used noun, verb, and modifier was checked against the cards and if the mother under assessment had not used that word before, a new card with the new word was added to her deck.

In the above manner, we could compute a "rarity index" for each noun, verb, and modifier, depending on the frequency with which it was used in our group of subjects. For example, if only one mother had used the word *travel*, she would have received a score of 42; if two mothers had used this word, each mother would have received a score of 41. Having thus translated the infrequency of usage into numbers, where the greater number represented a more unusual or rich use of language *relative to this group,* we could simply add each mother's richness score for nouns, verbs, and adjectives. Richness scores intercorrelated as follows: nouns and verbs .77; nouns and modifiers .68; verbs and modifiers .64. All three correlations were significant beyond the .01 level. For this reason we pooled the three richness scores into one, by taking a mean of the three for each subject.

Another linguistic measure was the number of compound sentences on every third page of the interview.

A third measure of language quality was that of overall grammatical competence. For any one of ten examples of good grammar the mother received one score (+1); for any one of five instances of bad grammar, she was given − 1. The total was her grammatical competence score.*

The correlation between compound sentences and grammatical competence was .69 ($p < .01$); thus these were averaged and each was taken as a measure of the quality of syntax.

In addition to the *richness of vocabulary* and the *syntax scores* we also had the length of the interview (range 33–120 typed pages), which we used as a measure of *talkativeness* in interaction with an adult.

With regard to the infant, we used the total Bayley Mental and Motor scores. Three verbal scores were created by William King and Bonnie Seegmiller, members of the project. Suspecting that many verbal items did not require verbal comprehension, King and Seegmiller defined Bayley Verbal Comprehension as follows: beginning with item 107 (puts beads in box: 6 of 8) and ending with item 163 (understands three prepositions), 40 items were judged to require the comprehension of verbal information for passing. The babies' Verbal Comprehension score was simply the number of such items passed.

Bayley Verbal Production scores were defined as follows: beginning with item 85 (says "da, da") and ending with item 150 (names watch), 16 items were judged as requiring the production of speech or talk. Items requiring both comprehension and production were counted with those requiring production.

In addition, King and Seegmiller used the raw score of the Uzgiris-Hunt Vocal Imitation Scale (Uzgiris & Hunt, 1969.)

---

*Examples of good grammar are tenses other than simple present or past (*had completed*), either–or constructions, and use of reflexives. Examples of bad grammar are run-on sentences, sentence fragments, slang terms, nonspecific nouns (*thing, stuff*).

We are grateful to Nancy Kalish-Landon, Ph.D. (Department of Psychology, California State University at Sacramento, Sacramento, California, 95819) who served as Research Assistant while a graduate student at the City University, for helping us develop these measures and quantifying the verbal data in the above manner.

*Readers with special interest in these Bayley and Hunt scores relative to language should contact

The hypothesis regarding the relationship of talkativeness, richness of vocabulary, and syntax to Bayley scores at three points in time was that only talkativeness and syntax will show a significant relationship to any of the Bayley scores. It was reasoned that of the three verbal measures derived from the interview, the mothers' syntactical sophistication would come closest to a measure of intelligence with possible relevance to cognitive development of the sons. Her talkativeness was seen as a sign of expressiveness and it was thought that expressive mothers would more likely be emotionally stimulating and may therefore have brighter sons.

Tables 4 and 5 present the results pertaining to this hypothesis.

Table 4.   Correlations Between Aspects of Maternal Language (Interview) and Infant Intelligence Scores (Bayley Scales) at 14, 18 and 22 Months

	Bayley Mental Scale			Bayley Motor Scale		
Aspects of Maternal Language	14 mos $n=42$	18 mos $n=31$	22 mos $n=29$	14 mos $n=42$	18 mos $n=31$	22 mos $n=29$
Talkativeness	.02	−.06	.06	.07	.08	−.08
Richness of vocabulary	.08	.18	.26	.04	−.03	−.02
Syntax	.09	.22	.25	−.05	.05	−.17

Table 5.   Correlations Between Aspects of Maternal Language (Interview) and Infants' Verbal Productivity, Verbal Comprehension (Bayley Scales), and Vocal Responsiveness Scores (Uzgiris-Hunt Scales) at 14, 18, and 22 Months

	Bayley Verbal Productivity			Bayley Verbal Comprehension			Uzgiris-Hunt Vocal Responsiveness		
Aspects of Maternal Language	14 mo $n=42$	18 mo $n=31$	22 mo $n=29$	14 mo $n=42$	18 mo $n=31$	22 mo $n=29$	14 mo $n=42$	18 mo $n=33$	22 mo $n=30$
Talkativeness	.13	.12	.00	.09	−.06	−.00	.21	.09	.36 [a]
Richness of vocabulary	.05	.30	.16	.18	−.01	.21	.07	.23	.28
Syntax	.13	.39 [a]	.34	.15	.03	.13	.06	.32 [a]	.17

[a] $p < .05$, two tailed.

William King, Department of Psychology, The City College of the City University of New York, 138th Street and Convent Avenue, New York, N.Y. 10031, for more detailed information.

The relationships between talkativeness, richness of vocabulary, and syntax to the total Bayley scores are eloquently insignificant, leaving no doubt about the appropriateness of accepting the null hypothesis. Not so when it comes to the three verbal scores derived by King and Seegmiller. Table 5 shows that both Bayley Verbal Productivity and Uzgiris-Hunt Vocal responsiveness relate significantly to maternal syntax level, as derived from the interview obtained when the infant was 14 months old. In other words, maternal syntax appears as a good candidate for predicting sons' verbal and vocal *output* at 18 months of age.

Table 5 also shows that maternal talkativeness (in the interview situation) may be a predictor of Vocal Responsiveness at 22 months of age. These correlations are low; nevertheless, they are significant beyond the .05 level of probability. Thus, we are not justified in declaring maternal talkativeness to an adult and syntactical sophistication as irrelevant in predicting verbal output at 18 and 22 months. The hypotheses stand confirmed except for the total Bayley scores as target data.

The reader will recall that maternal talking to the infant was double coded in the home observation scheme and that earlier its discussion was tabled. How much the mother talks to the infant in the home becomes relevant here, as we focus on her talking in relation to his cognitive development. The maternal language variables in Tables 4 and 5 were derived from the interview, where she was talking with another adult about her baby, but not to him, or in his presence. Let us then bring in the "mother talks" variable of the home observations at three points in time.

We may pose the question: of what might maternal talkativeness (to the interviewer when the baby was 14 months old and to the baby at 14, 18, and 22 months) be a predictor? Among the intercorrelations of maternal talkativeness, amount of chatting with the baby at 18 and 22 months of age relate most: $r = .64$; $n = 38$; $p < .01$, two-tailed test. The same variable shows an $r = .49$; $n = 43$; $p < .01$, two-tailed test, indicating somewhat less consistency of maternal behavior between 14 and 18 months than between 18 and 22 months of age. The amount of maternal talk with baby at 14 months of age shows an insignificant relationship to how much she will be talking to him at 22 months of age: $r = .21$; $n = 38$, n.s.—yet even this correlation is in the positive direction.

Is there any relationship between how much a mother talks to an adult interviewer *about* the baby and how much she talks *to* him at various times between 14 and 22 months? The correlations show that amount of maternal talk about the baby (when he was 14 months old) might be a better predictor than it is a correlate of the amount of talk to him: r's are .01, .29, and .30 at 14, 18, and 22 months, respectively, the latter two being significant beyond the

.01 level (n's are 43, 37, and 35, respectively). However, the modest size of these correlations cautions us against any assumption of a general talkativeness measure for mothers of infants, leaving open the possibility that as children become older and start to talk themselves, the relationship among maternal talkativeness measures might increase.

Having discarded the likelihood of a general talkativeness tendency in the mother, we can now ask an earlier question from another vantage point: Does the amount of maternal talk to the infant explain any variance of the Bayley scores (Mental and Motor) or of the Verbal Productivity, Comprehension or Responsiveness scores derived by King and Seegmiller? Tables 6 and 7 present the results.

Generally, the amount of talk with the infant in the home fares well as a correlate, pre-, and in some cases, post-dictor of variations in cognitive level among the infants. Table 6 shows that as far as total Bayley scores are concerned, the significant relationships concentrate on the Mental Scale. Amount of maternal talk at 14 months emerges as a predictor of the Bayley Mental Score at 22 months. Amount of maternal talk is correlated with the Mental Score at 18 months but does no better than the syntax measure taken from the interview. This variable is also a predictor from 18 to 22 months ($r = .41$; $df = 30, p < .02$) and is a correlate of the Bayley Mental score at 22 months. The post-dicting is about as good as the predicting: babies who measure higher at 14 months have mothers who talk more to them at 18 and 22 months of age. Since all the correlations in Table 6 regarding the Mental Scale are in the positive direction, and several fail to reach significance only by dint of a few missing degrees of freedom, it seems best to suggest a rather general conclusion: The amount of talking on the part of the mother is significantly implicated in the infant's cognitive development in the second year of life. That post-diction is almost as good as prediction may mean that babies contribute importantly by way of *eliciting* maternal talk.*

DOES PSYCHOLOGICAL MINDEDNESS IN MOTHERS EXPLAIN VARIATIONS IN INFANT INTELLIGENCE?

We propose that an important aspect of the mother's personality is the terms in which she thinks of the nature of her infant. In our pilot interviews we were struck by variations among mothers: some thought of the infant as primarily

---

*The reader will note the prevalence of two-tailed tests of significance throughout this report. The following section will see the use of one-tailed tests of significance (Tables 10 and 11, below). One-tailed tests were used where predictions were made with strong conviction arising from pilot data.

Table 6. Correlations Between "Mother Talks to Infant" (Home Observations) and Infant Intelligence Scores (Bayley Scales) at 14, 18, and 22 Months

Mother Talks to Infant	Bayley Mental Scale				Bayley Motor Scale		
	14 mo	18 mo	22 mo		14 mo	18 mo	22 mo
14 months	.21	.22	.33[a]		.12	.20	− .07
	$n=49$	$n=34$	$n=32$		$n=49$	$n=34$	$n=32$
18 months	.37[b]	.12	.36[c]		.22	.26	.04
	$n=42$	$n=34$	$n=32$		$n=42$	$n=34$	$n=32$
22 months	.48[d]	.41[b]	.38[c]		.29[a]	.08	.17
	$n=37$	$n=32$	$n=32$		$n=37$	$n=32$	$n=32$

[a] $p < .10$, two tailed.
[b] $p < .02$, two tailed.
[c] $p < .05$, two tailed.
[d] $p < .01$, two tailed.

Table 7. Correlations Between "Mother Talks to Infant" (Home Observations) and Infants' Verbal Productivity, Verbal Comprehension (Bayley Scales) and Vocal Responsiveness Scores (Uzgiris-Hunt Scales) at 14, 18, and 22 Months

Mother Talks to Infant	Bayley Verbal Productivity			Bayley Verbal Comprehension			Uzgiris-Hunt Vocal Responsiveness		
	14 mo	18 mo	22 mo	14 mo	18 mo	22 mo	14 mo	18 mo	22 mo
14 months	.27[a]	.18	.24	.30[b]	.20	.25	.26[a]	.01	−.04
	$n=49$	$n=34$	$n=32$	$n=49$	$n=34$	$n=32$	$n=51$	$n=36$	$n=33$
18 months	.25	.13	.33[a]	.34[b]	.09	.31[a]	−.04	.35[b]	.23
	$n=42$	$n=34$	$n=32$	$n=42$	$n=34$	$n=32$	$n=42$	$n=34$	$n=32$
22 months	.28[a]	.32[a]	.41[c]	.35[b]	.36[b]	.27	−.09	.37[b]	.39[b]
	$n=37$	$n=32$	$n=32$	$n=37$	$n=32$	$n=32$	$n=37$	$n=34$	$n=33$

[a] $p < .10$.
[b] $p < .05$.
[c] $p < .02$.

a *physical reality,* others conceived of him as a *psychological reality.* Still others did not supply us with data relevant to this.

To elaborate, some mothers portrayed the infant as one might a little animal who needs to be fed, changed, and housebroken. The only change they saw in their son since birth was that he became larger, and therefore heavier to carry around, had little idea of what developmental capabilities or limitations he had, or they had rather inappropriate ideas of what one might expect from a 14 month old. We noted their helpless submission to the child's will as though his perpetual motion just had to be tolerated until he wore himself out and fell asleep.

Other mothers perceived his psychological needs for security and stimulation, and noted his responsiveness to the moods of caretakers, including themselves. Such feeding or sleeping problems as they reported were cast in a psychological frame of reference. There was a general understanding that changes in circumstance affect the child's state and that he, in turn, could elicit reactions from others. They were impressed, at times enchanted, by the many changes in the first year of life and saw behavior as alterable by various teaching techniques. There was an understanding of themselves as agents of change, for example in regulating the infant's excitement level to avert temper tantrums.

We began to talk of such differences among the mothers as degrees of *psychological mindedness* and decided to devise a technique to elicit data from each mother relevant to it. We defined psychological mindedness along three continua: the mother's affective responsiveness to the infant, and her concept of developmental change and of behavior shaping. Ten critical incidents were selected from the pilot interviews to obtain relevant data from all mothers, even those whose interviews were otherwise constricted or shallow.

The hypothesis under test was that there will be significant positive correlations between mothers' psychological mindedness scores obtained at the outset of the study and Bayley Scale scores at 14, 18, and 22 months. The hypothesis thus expressed a parallel-diction and two predictions.*

The Method of Measuring Psychological Mindedness

Each of the ten critical incidents selected from pilot interviews states a situation in which mothers of infants in the second year of life often find themselves. Each requires some kind of evaluation, decision, and action. Upon hearing the interviewer describe a critical incident, most mothers begin immediately to reply, reflect, or associate to something that has recently happened with their

*The first author wishes to acknowledge her indebtedness to the late Helen D. Sargent of the Menninger Foundation who first discussed the concept of psychological mindedness in relation to the outcome of psychotherapy with adults. For the psychoanalytic formulation and research applications of this concept in other contexts see Wallerstein, Robbins, and Sargent (1956); Waldhorn (1967); Namnum (1968); Applebaum (1970). For a use in research concerning teacher–pupil relationships see Hill (1964).

baby that was similar to what the critical incident brings to mind. Following are examples of the critical incidents:

This baby used to be very friendly. He knew the people next door, some of his relatives, and also knew the man in the store. But one day he would have nothing to do with them, hid his face when he saw them, and wasn't friendly at all. Or,

This baby didn't want his mother to go out, and always wanted to be near her, and he wouldn't stay with anyone else, and wouldn't make up with anyone else. Or,

This baby's mother decided to feed him. She put him on her lap and began to give him some food. Suddenly, he didn't want it, threw it on the floor and began to cry.

Following each of ten such critical incidents mothers are asked to say why they think the baby might act this way and what action might a mother take. The responses are then detached and coded to disrupt a possible halo effect.

Each response is scored on three seven-point scales, where each of the seven points is defined. *The Affective Responsiveness Scale* reflects the degree to which the mother recognizes that babies' moods are variable and that there may be several emotional reasons for behavior. High scorers tend to consider the total situation, especially the context provided by the mother. *The Scale of Developmental Change* reflects the degree of understanding of age or stage appropriateness, even if the word "stage" is never used. High-scoring mothers show an understanding that time alone brings some alteration in babies' behavior or, at least, that the age or stage of the child has to be part of the judgment made by the mother about what is to be done. *The Scale for Behavior Shaping* reflects the mother's understanding that behavior can be molded or influenced by her through a variety of methods, none of which is likely to work on a single try. The overall PM Score is the mean of scores of each of ten responses on each of three seven-point scales.*

Table 8 shows that the intercorrelations among the three psychological mindedness scales justify pooling the scores and using the mean PM score for some purposes. The intercorrelations cannot exceed the interjudge reliabilities, which were in the high .80s and .90s for various pairs of judges.

It is important to point out that high interjudge reliability exists provided that judges' backgrounds are fairly homogeneous, for example, clinical psychologists working with children. Judges have to understand and accept the instructions and not make inferences *beyond* the scale-point definitions. For

---

*The instructions and full set of items together with scoring instructions may be obtained from the first author. (The Psychological Center, City College of the City University of New York, 3332 Broadway, New York, N.Y. 10031) These materials are now being used in various projects and have been found to be useful not only with mothers but also with day care center personnel in training. (Copyright applied for.)

Table 8.   Intercorrelations of Three Scales of Psychological Mindedness in Mothers of 14-Month-Old Infants ($N=40$)

Affective Responsiveness	Concept of Developmental Change	Concept of Behavior Shaping	Mean Psychological Mindedness
Affective responsiveness	.49[a]	.83[b]	.89[b]
Concept of developmental change		.57[b]	.74[b]
Concept of behavior shaping			.89[b]

[a] $p < .01$, two tailed.
[b] $p < .001$, two tailed.

example, in the pilot study two psychoanalyst raters agreed with each other but not with clinical psychologists working with young children. These raters again agreed with each other but not with one person trained primarily in education. Reliability here resides very much in the habits of thought of the rater and is not an abstract property of the instrument.

The PM score is then the mean of ten scores on three seven-point scales. Its mean for 46 mothers is 3.37 with an obtained range of 2.10–5.13, in the possible range of 1.00–7.00.

Before turning to additional statistical properties of the measure of psychological mindedness, as well as to results bearing on the hypothesis, two case samples will be presented in order to give the reader a *sense of the quality* of these data.

Case Illustrations of Psychological Mindedness

Timmy's mother's PM score was 2.27. Timmy's Bayley Mental Score plummeted from 116 at 14 months to 76 at 22 months. Johnny's mother's PM score was 5.13. Johnny's Bayley Mental Score was 116 at 14 months and rose to 120 by 22 months. (Both babies had above average Motor Scores which did not change.) Now let us look at how these mothers responded to the separation item above:

Timmy's mother: (laughs) Sometime it's too late to do anything. It is very hard to do anything with a spoiled baby, and it's bad on the mother too. Like, for instance, you could never go anywhere. Imagine me trying to go out at night, got to drag along the baby. It becomes very annoying because I don't feel as though a baby should interfere with the mother's social life either. I figure all that should fit in and so I think the mother is wrong . . . for letting the baby get that way. And see, I am lucky because my baby never got to that point where he actually never wanted to part with me . . .

stay by his side, nothing like that. He would cry if you leave him. Or he want you to hold him all the time, but other than that I never had that kind of problem.

Johnny's mother: He was just unfriendly, . . . well, kids, . . . that's also something that some babies I know, . . . Like I experienced it myself and Johnny wouldn't stay with anyone else, he'd cry and I felt at that particular time that he had a need to be with me whatever the reason was, and so I, you know, let him stay with me and after a while, you know, when he got to the stage when he felt confident, . . . and you know, everything worked out all right . . . I didn't know why. I wondered why he felt so secure, but then he was young, and since he was a young baby, you know, I accepted. Now if it had continued then it would have been worse. I felt that it was something I was doing, but my own theory worked out and that was, you know, that was it.

While Timmy's mother claims that she "never had that kind of problem," she believes it would have been gross interference in the mother's life. Johnny's mother reports problems around separation and that she felt " . . . at that particular time he had a need to be with me, whatever the reason was . . . " She struggles with the concept of "security" in him, showing that she does think in such affective and relational terms when she thinks of him. Note the readiness with which she considers that the separation problems might have had its roots in "something I was doing."

Items, Scales and Judgments; Some Properties of the Method

It will be recalled that while 44 mothers gave us interviews that were usable in their entirety, 46 mothers responded to the ten critical incidents administered as part of the interview. (Equipment failure made transcription of some interviews impossible, while the portions pertaining to psychological mindedness could be heard sufficiently well.) Thus the N for this part of the study is 46.

Taking the overall PM scores of 46 mothers, we asked several questions regarding the properties of the method itself. Since 25 mothers were administered the first five and 21 of the mothers the last five critical incidents first, we could test for possible order effect. We could also address ourselves to the question: do order, items, or scales have differential "pull" for high psychological mindedness?

A three-factor repeated-measures analysis of variance design was used with order of administration of critical incidents (two orders), between subjects, within subjects, between items (ten items), and scales of judgment (three scales) serving as variables. This is Winer's (1962) three-factor design with repeated measures on two factors, allowing for unequal n (unweighted means solution).*

*We are grateful to Richard Monahan, Ph.D. for suggesting this method.

Table 9 reveals that there is no significant order effect on the mothers' total PM scores, neither is there an order by item interaction, nor is there a scale by order interaction. There is, however, a significant item effect, in that one item "pulls" more psychological mindedness than the other nine. There is also a significant scale effect; at least one scale elicits higher psychological minded-ness than the other two. There is a significant item by scale interaction but no significant order by item by scale interaction.

Table 9.   Analysis of Variance; Three-Factor Design with Repeated Measurements on Two of the Factors and Unequal N, Regarding Psychological Mindedness Scores Depending on Items ($N=10$), Order of Administration ($N=2$), and Scales of Clinical Judgement ($N=3$) (subject $N=46$)

Source of Variance	Sum of Squares	Degrees of Freedom	Mean Squares	F	Significance Level
Between subjects	810.86	45			
Regular order[a]	3.43	1	3.43		
Subjects within groups (error variance)	807.45	44	18.35	.187	n.s.
Within subjects	3631.33	1334			
Items	121.46	9	13.50	5.32	$p < .01$
Order $\times$ items	32.88	9	3.65	1.44	n.s.
Items $\times$ subjects within groups (error variance)	1007.00	396	2.54		
Scales of judgment	860.69	2	430.35	131.61	$p < .01$
Order $\times$ scales	4.11	2	2.06	.63	n.s.
Scales of judgment $\times$ subjects within groups (error variance)	287.45	88	3.27		
Items $\times$ scales of judgment	184.69	18	10.26	8.27	$p < .01$
Order $\times$ items $\times$ scales of judgment	29.68	18	1.65	1.33	n.s.
Items $\times$ scales of judgment $\times$ subjects within groups (error variance)	984.22	792	1.24		

[a] Regular order of administration items 1–10 was compared with administering items 6–10 first and 1–5 last.

Which item and which scale "pull" higher scores can be determined only by inspection, which at this level of initial work with a small and select group of subjects seems unwarranted. These properties of the instrument do mean, however, that there is no reason to drop any of the ten items, nor any of the three scales, in order to shorten the task of assessment. This provisional stance toward the instrument is further strengthened by the results of *Duncan's*

Multiple Range Test (Edwards, 1968), a multiple comparison of individual items collapsed over the three scales: affective responsiveness, developmental change, and behavior shaping. Inspection of the table of intercorrelations among the ten items shows that items seven and ten differ significantly from items one and two and six. These items concern separation and exploratory behavior incidents (numbers seven and ten, respectively), while numbers one, two, and six concern eating and sleeping incidents. This makes clinical sense, and does not in itself justify discarding any of the ten critical incidents.

THE RELATIONSHIP OF PSYCHOLOGICAL MINDEDNESS IN MOTHERS AND COGNITIVE DEVELOPMENT OF THEIR INFANT SONS

To restate, the hypothesis under test was: There will be a significant and a positive correlation between psychological mindedness in mothers assessed at the time their sons are 14 months old, and the babies' cognitive development (a) as measured by the Bayley Mental scales and (b) as measured by the Bayley Motor scales. Tables 10 and 11 summarize the results.

Table 10.   The Relationship Between Psychological Mindedness in Mothers of 14-Month-Old Boys and Bayley Mental Scales of Infant Development at 14, 18, and 22 Months

Age	Psychological Mindedness Scales			
	Affective Responsiveness	Concept of Developmental Change	Concept of of Behavior Shaping	Mean Psychological Mindedness
14 months $N=46$	.24	.31[a]	.20	.33[a]
18 months $N=33$	.16	.28	.04	.22
22 months $N=32$	.46[c]	.44[b]	.35[a]	.46[c]

[a] $p < .05$, one tailed.
[b] $p < .02$, one tailed.
[c] $p < .001$, one tailed.

Note that the significant correlations at 14 months linking the mother's understanding of developmental changes and her entire PM score to the baby's cognitive development are significant but low ($r = .33$; $n = 46$; $p < .05$,

Table 11.   The Relationship Between Psychological Mindedness in Mothers of 14-Month-Old Boys and Bayley Motor Scales of Infant Development at 14, 18, and 22 Months

| | Psychological Mindedness Scales | | | |
Age	Affective Responsiveness	Concept of Developmental Change	Concept of Behavior Shaping	Mean Psychological Mindedness
14 months $N=46$	.40[b]	.05	.27[a]	.34[a]
18 months $N=33$	.22	.02	.18	.20
22 months $N=32$	.15	−.26	−.10	.01

[a] $p < .05$, one tailed.
[b] $p < .001$, one tailed.

one-tailed test). These correlations account for a very small amount of the variance. The prediction regarding the 18-months-old scores is insignificant. However, by the time the babies are 22 months old, psychological mindedness in mothers assessed 8 months before is statistically significant regarding all scales and climbs beyond the .001 level for her affective responsiveness as well as her total PM score ($r =. 46$; $n = 32$; $p < .001$, one-tailed test).

Only 3 out of 12 correlations in Table 11 reach significance, suggesting that the Motor Scales of the Bayley Test are much more independent of the mothers' personalities than the Mental Scales. One of these significant correlations is again with affective responsiveness, suggesting that perhaps for prediction (or parallel-diction, as in this case) affective responsiveness might turn out to be the most powerful scale of the three.

Let us focus on the correlation of .46 between PM scores from maternal data at 14 months and Bayley Mental Scale scores at 22 months. One views it with ambivalence. After all, it explains only 21% of the variance on the Bayley, yet this correlation emerged as a test of a hypothesis based on pilot data. It is not an adventitious result, and correlations of even this magnitude are seldom found with infant test data. The matter deserves serious consideration; in our caution not to clutter the literature with Type 1 errors, we must also avoid walking past a possible predictor of performance on Bayley Mental Scales and thus commit a Type 2 error.

To check on the possibility that the increasingly high r's with age were due only to selective attrition of subjects (loss of 14 subjects between 14 and 22 months), the correlations for the Mental Scale were recomputed for 14, 18, and 22 months, using only the 27 mother–infant pairs on whom all data were complete. Numerically, the correlations were higher than for the entire sample; however, the levels of significance were somewhat lower, no doubt because of loss of degrees of freedom. The r's for the 27 complete-data subjects at 14, 18, and 22 months were .42, $p < .02$; .31; n.s.; .38, $p < .02$, all one-tailed tests. Note that again we could explain none of the Bayley variance at 18 months, but some at 14 and 22 months, suggesting that the results in Table 10 cannot be attributed to selective attrition of subjects.

In evaluating the meaning of the possible parallel-dictive (14 months) and predictive (22 months) value of the psychological mindedness measure, we have also to address ourselves to the relationship of maternal language to it. After all, the responses are verbal, and it is entirely expectable that more verbal mothers would be judged as scoring higher.

Recall that maternal talkativeness and richness of vocabulary and syntax (in talking to an adult) explained none of the variance on total Bayley scores (Table 4) and that only syntactical sophistication predicted the infant's verbal productivity and vocal responsiveness and did so only at 18 months of age (Table 5). Recall also that the amount of talking to the infant in the home at 14 months related to the Bayley Mental scores, and appeared as a possible predictor from 14 to 22 months, that is, the amount of maternal talk to the infant at 14 months related to his Bayley Mental score at 22 months ($r - .48$; n-37; $p < .01$, two tailed). Generally, talking to the infant fared well as a correlate and even as a post-dictor (Tables 6 and 7).

Relevant to maternal talk and psychological mindedness, we have to conclude that while measures of the sophistication of her language in a dialogue with an adult relate considerably to psychological mindedness, *unlike the relation to Bayley scores,* the amount she talks to her baby relates not at all to psychological mindedness, *unlike the relation to Bayley scores.* Table 12 reveals that there is no sense thinking of psychological mindedness independent of the ability to express oneself to the interviewer, but that talking to baby is unrelated to such psychological mindedness.

In conclusion, the hypothesis that psychological mindedness explains a significant amount of variance on the Bayley Scales is upheld for the Mental Scale at 14 and 22 months, and for the Motor Scale at 14 months. Methodological explorations suggest that the critical incidents do elicit responses that can then be reliably scored according to three scales. Results of a three-factor repeated analysis of variance test give no reason to suspect an order effect and caution against reducing either the number of items or scales of judgment.

Table 12.   Correlations Between Psychological Mindedness Scales and Several Measures of Maternal Language

Measures of Maternal Language	Measures of psychological mindedness			
	Affective Responsiveness	Concept of Developmental Change	Concept of Behavior Shaping	Mean Psychological Mindedness
Measures derived from interview (N=43):				
Talkativeness	.35[b]	.25[a]	.45[d]	.39[c]
Richness of vocabulary	.48[d]	.35[b]	.42[d]	.44[d]
Syntax	.41[d]	.31[b]	.48[d]	.45[d]
Measure derived from home observations:				
Talks to infant				
14 mo (N=46)	.03	.06	.18	.09
18 mo (N=40)	.07	.23	.20	.26
22 mo (N=37)	.17	.03	.09	.22

[a] $p < .10$, two tailed.
[b] $p < .05$, two tailed.
[c] $p < .02$, two tailed.
[d] $p < .01$, two tailed.

DISCUSSION

This report initiates the integration of data collected from a group of Black male infants and their mothers, from three vantage points (infant tests, home observations, and maternal interviews) over an 8-month period in the second year of life. The three-pronged investigation was stimulated by a need for description of the life circumstances of mothers and their first-born sons in an urban ghetto. In addition there was the need to answer two specific questions: (1) Schaefer (1969) reported that cognitive functioning in his own subjects as well as in subjects from other studies deteriorated with age, in the second year of life. Was this also true of the infants we tested? (2) Do interpersonal and situational variables covary with cognitive development in the second year of life?

Throughout we provided various descriptions, portraits of mothers, and home observation impressions that suggest a surprising amount of variation in caretaking attitudes and living arrangements as well as environments surrounding (and affecting) our group of infants. This means that no matter how homogeneous a black infant sample from an urban ghetto may be with regard

o variables pertaining to the infants alone, one might expect powerful be-
ween-infant differences in all other areas. Future studies designed to explore
he fate of cognition may benefit from further descriptive work, extending the
imits of understanding to a greater degree of specificity of the relevant dimen-
ions of life circumstances. While some of these dimensions such as maternal
alkativeness and emotional responsiveness may be affected by characteristics
f the infant himself, others are likely to exist prior to his birth, or are clearly
eyond his "sphere of influence."

Similarly, the varieties of caretaking arrangements merit further study.
Mothers in urban ghettos find many kinds of solutions to the problems of
caretaking, involving grandmothers, other family members, and paid sitters.
These adults orbit around the infants in many ways, appearing at various times
luring the day and the week. We cannot yet speak to the long-range effects
nd correlates of these patterns of care. Nevertheless, we wish to raise the
question of whether the seven caretaking patterns we identified earlier would
ccount for all detectable variations in a larger, randomly selected sample. (In
Table 1 we defined five patterns of primary caretaking by the biological mother
nd two patterns of care in which she plays a minor role.) The definition of
a finite set of patterns of care could then lead to a study of their "anatomy."
This, in turn, would surely deepen our understanding of how adults arrange
hemselves around infants, how the orbit of females moves and rearranges
tself in time around a growing male child. Not only the store of knowledge
f the field of child development but also planners of intervention programs
would benefit from a systematic study of caretaking patterns. These are numer-
us, relevant, and knowable.

Turning now to the question of cognitive deterioration, recall that this has
een dealt with elsewhere by King and Seegmiller (1973), and summarized in
he present paper. Briefly, in this context, the fate of the Bayley Scale scores
lo not permit the conclusion that black infants *in general* fall below the United
States norms by 22 months of age. The mean of 107 at 14 months declines to
00 by 22 months. The Bayley Mental Scale scores of first-born black male
nfants (selected as described earlier) *does* decline in the second year of life but
not below population norms. This result leaves us with several possibilities.
Clearly, this sample was a superior one; the above-average mean score at 14
months is easy to explain by the method of selection, which eliminated from
he study any infant with questionable health. The decline could be a regres-
ion toward the mean. It could also be that at this early age deprived environments act the same way upon average and above-average infants. Such specula-
ions are tempered by the fact that individual drops of 40 and gains of 25 points
vere found. In a relatively small sample changes of such magnitude deflect
rom the importance of the fate of mean scores and underline the importance

of the study of correlates. As in the case of the varieties of caretaking patterns, so here: increased understanding of the correlates of large shifts in level of cognitive development within a short, yet critical period of time is needed not only from a general scientific point of view but also for the planning of intervention programs. Clearly, an infant whose Bayley Mental score plummets by 40 points in 8 months requires different "early intervention" from another one who maintains his average status, or still another one who climbs into the upper 10% of the population of infants. Where social planning exists but is not "good enough," such black infants may be the beneficiaries of the same "early intervention program" particularly if they live in the same health area!

Of the many interpersonal and situational correlates of the fate of cognitive development in the entire investigation, this paper focused on a few. Before discussing results pertaining to mother-infant relationship, let us recall that only 29 of 45 mothers were primary and only caretakers of the babies at the outset of the study. This fact stacks the cards against significant correlations, that is, in favor of the null hypothesis. Because the pilot study did not alert us to this possibility, we choose now to include in the analyses all good cases, even where mother–infant pairs have infrequent contact, thereby increasing the likelihood of Type 2 errors. We could, of course, eliminate such mother–infant pairs post facto, thereby working with an even more homogeneous sample, that is, only those with conventional and similar caretaking patterns, but then we would not know whether the reduced variation would result in reduced chances for significant correlations or whether the hypotheses based on the implicit assumption of primary caretaking by the natural mother would indeed be favored by the postfacto screening of subjects. In such a situation one chooses according to one's bent; in the end, we felt the postfacto elimination of subjects to be more suspect than any other tack we might have taken. These matters may be too obvious to belabor, yet, with regard to the further study of ghetto children there is here a caveat, hence the methodological problem posed by varieties of caretaking is highlighted. Clearly, future research must deal planfully with these patterns of caretaking, particularly where mother–infant relationships are being studied.

There certainly appear to be correlates as well as predictors of the fate of cognitive development in the second year of life. Those reported here pertain to the mother's behavior as well as to other personality attributes inferred by judges who were unaware of Bayley data. Below we summarize how different aspects of the mother relate to or predict cognitive development at 14, 18, and 22 months. Note the implicit assumption that the Bayley Scales provide a valid measure of the *quality of the infant;* a relatively precise but narrow-band assessment of the babies!

At 14 months, encouragement of performance by the mother that elicits an instrumental response from the baby relates positively to Bayley Mental scores while providing distraction and sedentary (soothing) stimulation relate negatively. The mother's talkativeness at this age explains none of the variance. Yet, in its relationship to Bayley Mental scores at 22 months of age, talkativeness at 14 months suggests itself as a predictor.

The maternal attribute of psychological mindedness correlates with both mental and motor scores at 14 months, as was hypothesized. By inspection, the Affective Responsiveness Scale of the three Psychological Mindedness Scales seems to pull most weight.

At 18 months, a mother present in the home, but occupied with matters other than the baby, that is, a psychologically unavailable mother, is likely to have a duller baby, while one who is available for imitative play is likely to have a brighter baby. Reward, punishment, and affectionate contact—all three kinds of behavior correlate with Bayley Motor Scale scores; .39, .49, .59 ($N = 34$) respectively. While these correlations do not explain spectacular amounts of variance, they are nevertheless large enough to command attention.

Also at 18 months, the mother's level of syntax relates to verbal productivity and vocal responsiveness of the infant. Eighteen months of age is the only time in the second year of life when the mother's syntax is at all relevant. The amount she talks to him at home relates to how vocally responsive he is. Her psychological mindedness is not a correlate of Bayley scores at 18 months.

Obviously, the aspects of the mother that are relevant to test performance are not the same at 14 as at 18 months. *How the mother feels about and thinks about the child covaries with his performance at 14 months, while what she does and that she does involve herself with him covary with aspects of cognitive measures at 18 months.* Note that at 18 months punishing explains as much variation in the positive direction ($r = .49; n = 34; p < .01$) as her unavailability explains in the negative direction ($r = -.49; n = 34; p < .01$). This suggests that the shift in the relationship requires more definitive, overt behavior from the mother at 18 months than at 14 months. This interpretation is in concert with the observation by King and Seegmiller (1973) that 18-month-old boys are much more difficult to test than are 14-month-old boys.

Correlations only delineate the area where causality might reside. Either brighter babies elicit more definite, overt behavior from the mother, or mothers who behave with greater clarity and interact more have brighter babies. It is also possible that these aspects of mothering as well as of infant performance are determined by other variables not studied here. But all reservations aside, the most parsimonious interpretation of the shifts from 14 to 18 months is that while affectionate aspects of mothering stay relevant, they do so in different modalities, and that, generally speaking, by 18 months of age maternal behav iors that are more like those of teachers emerge as significant in the relation ship. All this suggests the following hypothesis: if our aim is to increase cognitive competence, at 18 months of age teaching methods consisting o definite, comprehensible overt acts performed with maximum psychologica presence, accompanied by utterances in clear, concise sentences, will be mos effective. This hypothesis does not deny the importance of *affection* at this o at other ages, but it does imply (to use Bettelheim's words) that in the middl of the second year of life "love is not enough."

In contrast to earlier ages, by 22 months we have a better harvest of signifi cant and positive correlations between maternal and infant variables. Holding talking, imitating, and instructing covary with higher infant test scores. Dulle infants spend more time self-stimulating in the home. Psychological minded ness in mothers assessed at the outset of the study, when the infants were 1 months old, correlates .46 ($n = 32$; $p < .001$) with Bayley Mental scores a 22 months, and thus presents itself as a likely predictor of cognitive develop ment.

Mothers who talk more to their infants at home have brighter infant according to Bayley and Uzgiris-Hunt measures, and these mothers' talkative ness also relates to 18 months test scores. Since talkativeness to the infant doe not relate to psychological mindedness, we can consider these aspects of moth ering to be independent correlates of the infant test scores. This suggests tha there may be more than one way to a high mental test score at 22 months several behavioral aspects of the mother and at least one aspect that reflect how she construes her infant.

As in comparing 14 and 18 months results, so in comparing 18 and 22 months results we must conclude that different aspects of the mothers' atti tude, feelings, and behavior are relevant for cognitive development at differen times. Also it seems that within this 8-month period there is increasing evi dence for covariation between maternal and infant variables. This is a more conservative interpretation than King and Seegmiller's (1973) suggestion of ar "18-months effect."

Several explanations are possible. It could be that infant tests become more valid as infants get older, increasing the likelihood of significant correlations with maternal variables. This hypothesis could be tested in future studies where the *quality of the infant* would be measured by assessment technique that have a broader spectrum than infant tests.

It could also be that in these 8 months, infants become more psychologically integrated and that increased integration makes for more valid assessment and thus gives rise to more covariation with maternal variables.

We have also to consider that aspects of mothering require time to show cumulative impact in interaction with the baby; this interpretation is suggested by psychological mindedness having a greater predictive than parallel-dictive power. This explanation is similar to that of Kagan (1969), who reported that amount of babbling did not correlate with social class variables until 27 months of age. The kind of thinking required to score high on the Psychological Mindedness Scales requires trial action with regard to the baby, who is conceived of as separate and different from the mother. A certain degree of individuality of needs and propensities has to be perceived and appreciated in him. It may well be that a multitude of tacit communications from a psychologically minded mother enhance the separation-individuation process, which, according to Mahler (1969), is the primary developmental task in the second year of life.

Because the integration of data from three domains continues, and while previously unpublished results emerge in print (Wieder, 1972) and followup information is still being analyzed, it is premature to reach more definitive conclusions. Nevertheless, several comments pertaining to the method and structure of the investigation are in order, going beyond the data. We have opinions regarding applied clinical work with mothers and infants in circumstances similar to our subjects.

Studying the relationship between maternal verbal report and laboratory observation of mothers' teaching behavior, Hoenig, Tannenbaum, and Caldwell (1973) found that only 6 of 48 variables correlated significantly. This fact led the authors to express considerable pessimism about the possibility of finding convergence between what mothers say they do, and what they actually do. For several reasons we are not yet ready to agree. We have not placed mothers in a laboratory situation and recommend against it for several reasons. The young mother of a first-born is likely to feel very much under scrutiny and can be assumed to be more comfortable in her home. Were we to find relationships between teaching styles in a laboratory situation and what the mother reports about herself, we would still not know whether she does at home as she does in the laboratory. Because in the end all methods of assessment will have some effect of the subjects (mothers or babies), we recommend data collection from multiple vantage points and by independent teams. The problem of strategy is the *choice* of vantage points, and not whether to collect data about babies from more than one domain.

We do not know why certain mothers discontinued their participation in the study. There is some evidence that theirs were the less bright babies (King & Seegmiller, 1973), and an inspection of the length of the interviews reveals that women in the attrition group gave shorter interviews. While two research assistants and one project secretary were black, the project was initiated by and represented as the work of white investigators. The fact that a larger group of mothers chose to continue and even to resume contact several years later is no evidence against the possibility that many mothers might have felt more comfortable with a black staff. The paucity of black investigators leaves this question an open one for some time.

As to the implications of these results for planning intervention programs firm recommendations will have to await the completion of all work, including the followup study. Nevertheless, we are ready to conclude that not all black infants in an urban ghetto need intervention, early education, or any other kind of psycho-educational experience other than that which the mother provides. A large proportion of these mother–infant pairs are faring very well, sometimes in a conventional nuclear family, sometimes in a one-parent family, either with a fairly acceptable economic base, or in the face of tremendous social and economic handicaps. But there are others whose life circumstances and whose relationships with their infants forecast nothing but catastrophe. It is our impression that these are the youngest mothers and the ones whose own childhoods were foreshortened by early family disintegration and geographical dislocation. As one such 18-year-old mother said: "You want to know how I feel about my future? My future is behind me." Such varieties will be documented in forthcoming publications. At present, the portraits of three mothers offered earlier should give a glimpse of how soon mother–infant relationships coagulate and how various their quality.

One cannot work with mothers and infants in Harlem and not develop strong feelings about intervention; as the field notes of H. Nechin show, the impact upon the observer of that which is observed is considerable. Thus, even before one can fully substantiate one's convictions with data, one is given to form opinions about what all these results might in the end imply for social planning.

A recent review of the effects of early intervention studies (Lichtenberg & Norton, 1971) summarizes evidence from numerous studies. It is clear that short-term intervention studies result in higher mental test scores for children under 3 years of age and that mothers can be taught to better cope with them. However, gains evaporate once the studies are over and subjects are left to their own devices. The authors advocate long-term intervention programs and suggest that the earlier in the child's life they are put into operation, the more effective they are likely to be. We concur strongly. But, we wonder: how early is early enough?

In *Tomorrow's tomorrow,* Joyce A. Ladner (1971) gives a descriptive account of the social and psychological evolution of black girls. Many of the interview excerpts that document her conclusions could as well have come from our files. Since our mothers were an unusually young group, it is possible to cogwheel with Ladner's girls who also were poor and lived in urban centers.

It appears that pregnancy in the life of an adolescent black girl has, generally speaking, a positive value. Not that there are not black families who consider early pregnancy a mistake. But, from within the frame of reference of the girls themselves, pregnancy brings with it a "changed self-conception from one who was approaching maturity to one who had attained the status of womanhood"

(Ladner, 1971, p. 218). And elsewhere: "The anticipation of womanhood is symbolished . . . by belief by some of these preadolescents that having a baby will achieve a certain kind of responsibility for the girl, and consequent womanhood . . . acceptance of having a baby as a symbol of womanhood was expressed by girls of all ages" (p. 123).

Might it not be that a Headstart program for mothers during the adolescent years would be a more effective way of helping than intervention programs after birth or when the baby is 3 years of age? It would appear that the experience of caring for one's siblings—a responsibility many of our subjects carried while still children themselves—is not enough to prepare girls to be sufficiently effective in coping with their own babies, but that this child-caring experience would be of good use if it were coupled with some substantive learning of how babies grow, what their eating and sleeping patterns are like, that they can learn, that "strengthening the lungs" may not be the only consequence of letting an infant "cry it out," that clinging is natural, and that exploring the kitchen cupboards is good. Such cognitive preparation for motherhood might interdigitate with the increased self-valuing that pregnancy is said to bring to the black girl and could be said to be *preventive* not only because of the concern for the as yet unborn, but also because so many of the mothers are youngsters themselves.

REFERENCES

Ambrose, A. (Ed.), *Stimulation in early infancy.* New York: Academic Press, 1969.

Appelbaum, S.A. Psychological mindedness: Word, concept and essence. Paper delivered at the midwinter meeting of the American Psychoanalytic Association, New York, N.Y., 1970.

Bayley, N. *Bayley scales of infant development: Birth to two years.* New York: Psychological Corporation, 1969.

Bettelheim, B. *The empty fortress.* New York: Free Press, 1967.

Brown, R. *The first language.* Cambridge: Harvard University Press, 1974.

Caldwell, B. & Herscher, L. et al. Mother–infant interaction in monomatric and polymatric families. *American Journal Orthopsychiatry,* 1963, **33,** 653.

Edwards, A.L. *Experimental design in psychological research* (3rd ed.). New York: Holt, Rinehart and Winston, Inc., 1968, pp. 131–135.

Hill, E.L. The differential management of critical learning situations. (Unpublished Ed.D. thesis, Harvard Graduate School of Education, Cambridge, Mass., 1964).

Honig, M.A., Tannenbaum, J. & Caldwell, B.M. Maternal behavior in verbal report and in laboratory observation: a methodological study. *Child Psychiatry and Human Development,* 1973, **3** 216–230.

Joint Commission on Mental Health of Children. *Crisis in child mental health.* New York: Harper and Row, 1970.

Kagan, J. Some response measures that show relations between social class and the course of cognitive development in infancy. In A. Ambrose, (Ed.), *Stimulation in early infancy.* New York: Academic Press, 1969, pp. 253–257.

Kagan, J. & Moss, H.A. Parental correlates of child's IQ and height: a cross validation of the Berkeley Growth Study results. *Child Development,* 1959. **30,** 325–332.

King, W.L. & Seegmiller, B. Performance of 14 to 22 months old Black first born male infants on two tests of cognitive development. *Developmental Psychology,* 1973, **8** 317–326.

Ladner, J.A. *Tomorrow's tomorrow.* New York: Doubleday, 1971.

Lichtenberg, P. & Norton, D.G. Cognitive and mental development in the first five years of life. Rockville, Md., National Institute of Mental Health, Public Health Service Publ. No. 2057, 1971.

Lipsitt, L.P. The experiential origins of human behavior. In L. Goulet and P. Baltes (Eds.), *Life-span developmental psychology.* New York, Academic Press, 1970, pp. 285–303.

Mahler, M.S. *On human symbiosis and the vicissitudes of individuation.* New York: International University Press, 1968.

Moss, H.A. & Robson, N. Determinants of maternal stimulation of infants and the consequence of this treatment for later reactions to strangers (ms., 1969).

Namnum, A. The problem of analyzability and the autonomous ego. *International Journal of Psychoanalysis,* 1968, **49,** 254–275.

Olim, E.G. Maternal language styles and children's cognitive behavior. *Journal of Special Education,* 1970, **4,** 53–68.

Schaefer, E.S. Home tutoring, maternal behavior and infant intellectual development. Paper presented at the meeting of the American Psychological Association, Washington, D.C., September, 1969.

Spitz, R. *No and yes; on the genesis of human communication.* New York: International University Press, 1957.

Uzgiris, I.C. & Hunt, J.M. An instrument for assessing infant psychological development. University of Illinois Psychological Development Laboratory, Urbana, Author, 1966 (mimeo).

Waldhorn, H. *Indications for psychoanalysis.* New York, International University Press, 1967.

Wallerstein, R.S. et al. The psychotherapy research project of the Menninger Foundation; Concepts. *Bulletin of the Menninger Clinic,* 1956, **20,** 239–262.

Wieder, S. The texture of early maternal experience: maternal control and affect in relation to the second year of life. (Unpublished Ph.D. thesis, City University of New York, New York, N.Y., 1972).

Winer, B.J. *Statistical principles in experimental design.* New York: McGraw-Hill., 1962.

CHAPTER 2

Television and Personality Development: The Socializing Effects of an Entertainment Medium*

ROBERT M. LIEBERT AND RITA WICKS POULOS

When the first radio programs and the first films began to enjoy popularity among the young, they were immediately accused by critics of increasing delinquency rates while hailed by enthusiasts as bringing new culture and literacy, in palatable form, to millions of young for the first time (Bogart, 1972; DeFleur, 1970; Maccoby, 1964). So it has been with television.

But television is also different, in at least some respects. For one thing, the enormous amount of time viewers invest in the medium is virtually unprecedented for any entertainment form in history. When it was said of a child 30 years ago that he spent "all of his time" at the movies, the reference was usually to a Saturday morning cartoon and serial marathon at a local theater, embellished perhaps by one or two single features during the week; the latter luxury was enjoyed by only the children of the prosperous and those with particularly lucrative paper routes. Seven- and eight-year-old children were rarely seen huddling around a radio on pleasant summer afternoons instead of playing outside, and comic books were sought after as much because they could be

*The research reported in this paper was supported, in part, by grants from General Foods Corporation, General Mills, Inc., Lilly Endowment, Markle Foundation, National Institute of Child Health and Human Development, National Institutes of Mental Health, and United Methodist Communications; portions of the work were conducted at the Media Action Research Center, Inc., Nelson Price, President.

The Wrather Corporation generously provided the *Lassie* programs. Special thanks are due our colleagues for their valuable collaboration in carrying out the various projects: Elaine Brimer, Michael Cooney, Ann Covitz, Emily S. Davidson, Patricia Donagher, Francine Hay, Carol Keating, Marsha Liss, David Morgenstern, John M. Neale, Steven Schuetz, Jeannie Shu, Joyce N. Sprafkin, and Elanna Yalow.

collected and traded as because they could be read.

By way of contrast to these modest doses of earlier entertainment media, television captures the attention of nursery and elementary school-age children for an average of 3 hours per day, 7 days a week; by age 16, most children in the United States will have spent more time watching television than going to school (Liebert, Neale, & Davidson, 1973; Lyle & Hoffman, 1972). Saturation, too, is more complete for television than for any of its predecessors. A virtually unknown luxury in 1946, television can now be found in 98% of all American homes (See Figure 1)—more homes by far than have adequate heat or indoor plumbing. This spiraling saturation is found not only in the United States, but throughout the world. According to the United States Information Agency, as early as 1965 there were more than 20 million television sets in the Far East, an equal number in Eastern Europe, and nearly 7 million sets in Latin America and the Caribbean alone.

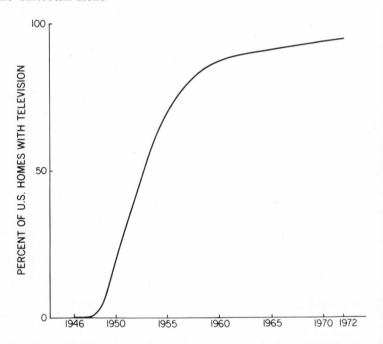

Figure 1.   Percentage of American homes with one or more television sets during the years 1946–1972. (Source: Based on data provided by Television Information Office.)

But while the United States rarely imports programs from abroad, save for the occasional BBC classic that achieves limited success on the lean and struggling airwaves of our Public Broadcasting System, American programming is seen by youngsters in heavy doses almost everywhere that television has taken hold; most often it consists of reruns of our most popular action-adventure and situation comedy shows, dubbed when economically feasible, and subtitled when necessary. About 40% of the programs seen in Japan and Formosa are American imports (Gardner, 1961; Tsai, 1969), as are nearly a third of the programs seen in Sweden, Great Britain, and Israel (Dahlgren, 1972; Halloran & Croll, 1972; Shinar, 1972). Even in Eastern Europe, American shows have a profound influence; the Polish Communist Party abandoned Wednesday night as a meeting time, so members could watch the popular *Dr. Kildare* (*Time*, 1968). In fact, a cross-national study by Robinson (1972) of 11 countries* indicated that television, across the board, " . . . appears to have had a greater influence on the structure of daily life than any other innovation in this century" (1972, p. 428).

What, if any, are the socializing effects of this massive diet of television entertainment upon the young? A hint is provided by investigations conducted in an earlier era, which supplied at least limited evidence that specific movies, comic books, and radio plays could significantly alter the attitudes and behavior of the young who were exposed to them (e.g., Peterson, Thurstone, Shuttleworth & May, 1933; Preston, 1941; Siegel, 1956, 1958; Zajonc, 1954).

In this chapter we outline the present state of our knowledge regarding television and personality development. While the review is by no means exhaustive, emphasizing as it does our own research and that of others also working within the social learning tradition, an effort has been made to capture the wide and growing edge of knowledge in the area and to relate theory and basic research to the applied, practical issues that arise in the social, economic, and political milieu in which commercial broadcasting decisions are made.

How are we to determine the possible effects of entertainment media interacting, as they certainly must, with a multitude of complementary and antagonistic influences emanating from the child's interaction with parents, peers, teachers, and the world at large? The relevant questions do not easily lend themselves to answers, but neither are they unique. The problems that arise in analyzing television's possible impact on children are quite similar to those encountered in trying to understand the role of other single input factors (e.g., the influence of parental warmth or peer modeling) in the overall process of socialization. We must look for converging and complementary information from established basic research and relate these segments of knowledge to a workable theoretical framework to assemble and analyze a variety of data regarding the interaction between media input and the child.

---

*Belgium, Bulgaria, Czechoslovakia, East Germany, France, Hungary, Peru, Poland, United States, West Germany, and Yugoslavia.

CONCEPTUALIZING MEDIA INFLUENCES: OBSERVATIONAL LEARNING

An analysis of the effects of exposure to television entertainment can be approached from different vantage points, but we believe the most useful starting point is the basic theoretical concept of observational learning. Specifically observational learning involves changes brought about in one person's (the observer's) behavior as a result of exposure to the actions of others (the models), either directly or symbolically through books, films, television, and the like. That children learn much about the world observationally is well established; the process has been demonstrated experimentally for language acquisition (e.g., Bandura & Harris, 1966; Liebert, Odom, Hill, & Huff, 1969) generalized forms of rule-learning (Zimmerman & Rosenthal, 1974), transmission of disciplinary practices (Walters, Leat, & Mezei, 1963), and sharing (e.g. Bryan & London, 1970; Rosenhan & White, 1967), to name only a few.

The Three Stages of Observational Learning

How exactly does observational learning take place? We have found it useful to conceptualize the process as involving three major stages (cf. Liebert, 1972, 1973): *exposure, acquisition,* and *acceptance* (See Figure 2).

For observational learning to occur the observer must first be exposed to the specific acts or modeling cues embodied in someone else's behavior. Exposure to a particular behavioral example can occur, however, without necessarily leading to learning or retention; a youngster may simply fail to comprehend or process what is being shown. Then, too, modeling cues may be misunderstood, in which case the enduring products of observational learning would be difficult to anticipate from inspection of the modeled bahavior alone.

The second stage of observational learning is therefore one of *acquisition,* including the comprehension, interpretation, and storage of what has been seen and heard. The study of acquisition processes has begun to enjoy a central role in the work of researchers concerned with the larger phenomenon of observational learning and is an important key to the often remarkably complex and sometimes subtle effects of television.

The third and final stage of observational learning is *acceptance;* does a child, having been exposed to modeling cues and having extracted information from them, now accept and assimilate the distilled content as a guide for his own subsequent actions?

Acceptance, of course, can take many forms. The simplest (and perhaps least common) manifestation of acceptance is to directly imitate or copy what one has seen or, obversely, to explicitly avoid performing a particular modeled behavior (that is, direct *counter*-imitation). The far more likely and com-

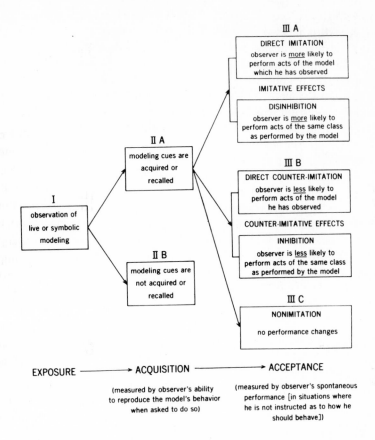

Figure 2. The three major stages involved in observational learning.

plicated acceptance effects that occur in observational learning involve generalizations—and transformations—on semantic and conceptual dimensions as well as concrete physical ones. Broad classes of behavior thus may potentially be inhibited or disinhibited through observational learning.

APPLICATION OF THE FRAMEWORK

The foregoing model, derived from basic studies of observational learning, serves as an outline for reviewing our knowledge of television's potential socializing effects, and also helps direct and refine the research path that lies ahead. For example, the framework's emphasis on exposure to specific classes of modeling cues leads to a search for full description of each viewer's exact TV diet and to detailed analyses of television content. Likewise, viewing the acquisition stage as an independent process that mediates the exposure–acceptance relationship demands studies of comprehension of televised material and emphasizes the possible importance of developmental factors as mediators of age-differentiated findings in overt behavior. And, finally, the framework leads to a broad-spectrum search for acceptance effects; narrow and simplistic dependent measures begin to yield to a multidimensional inspection of impact. As one example, the possible effects of violent content on television may extend well beyond an increased willingness by the observer to aggress, himself. Greater willingness to approve or tolerate the aggressive acts of others, a lowered sensitivity to real-life aggression, expectations of personal victimization, and decrements in cooperative behavior all are indirect manifestations of the original input (e.g., Dominick & Greenberg, 1972; Drabman & Thomas, 1974; Gerbner & Gross, 1974; Hapkiewicz & Roden, 1971).

Having outlined the theoretical framework we employ to organize and understand television's possible effects, we can now use it to examine data bearing on the role of television as an agent of socialization.

EXPOSURE

In considering the impact of television, the broadest question pertaining to exposure has to do with the degree to which the medium has pervaded the daily lives of children. We spoke to this issue earlier; most youngsters watch television at least 2–3 hours daily, and many watch twice that amount. Parents contribute to the heavy use of the medium by employing television as an "electronic babysitter"; by one estimate (Johnson, 1967) almost four-fifths of all American parents do so. What is more, although Saturday morning is children's "prime time" and therefore represents peak viewing for younger children, weekday evenings also are heavy viewing hours for children as well as their parents. Lyle and Hoffman (1972) found that 10–15% of a large sample of 7- and 8-year-old California youngsters were still watching television at 9:30 p.m. on weekdays. Turning to another survey, and a wider range of middle childhood, McIntyre and Teevan (1972) state: " . . . on one Monday during the period covered, over five million children under the age of 12 were still watching between 10:30 and 11:00 p.m. . . . "

To what content and lessons are children exposed during the many and various hours they sit in front of the television set? That question is the next one to which our analysis of exposure leads. No one study, to our knowledge, has tried to completely describe the content of a sample of television shows; rather, investigators have tended to select and analyze aspects of content pertinent to particular interests and issues. Our subsequent discussion is therefore topical, and should be introduced with the caution that we are crossing boundaries of time, sampling procedures, and specific definitions of content.

Agression and Violence

Indices of the amount of violence and aggression on television have appeared more regularly over the past two decades than measures of any other aspect of the medium's content. Definitionally, there has been considerable argument as to what these terms mean, but generally content analysts have emphasized actions that are harmful or potentially destructive to the person and property of others; a component of hostility may be present, but is not always implied inasmuch as instrumental aggression can clearly occur—on television and in life—without an affective component.

Violence and aggression could be found in some of the first television plays, just as they were present in the earliest radio shows and movies. Through the 1950s and 1960s, though, there was a shift from violence as *one* theme of television entertainment to violence as *the* theme of television entertainment. In 1954, for example, a relatively temperate 17% of prime time entertainment was devoted to "action-adventure" programming that emphasized gun-toting, two-fisted heroes who solved conflicts (and won inevitable victory) with overt force; by 1961 this figure had risen to 60% and by 1969 it had crossed the 80% mark (Gerbner, 1972; Liebert et al., 1973). According to a more recent analysis, attention to the related themes of violence and crime appear to have risen further in general programming during the 1969–1972 period (Gerbner, 1974, p. 73).

An aggressive or violent act, of course, does not occur in a vacuum, and so contextual information becomes as significant as simple frequency counts. Full analyses of context have yet to be done, but two facts stand out sharply: aggressive acts portrayed on television entertainment are usually shown as the most successful way of reaching goals (e.g., Stein, 1972) and the aggressor is most likely to be a white male (Donagher, Poulos, Liebert, & Davidson, 1975; Gerbner 1972). As a concrete illustration, consider a recent analysis in our laboratory of nine prime-time shows including both black and white characters in main roles. White males were engaged in almost two aggressive altercations over every 5 minutes of screen appearance; for the remaining groups (black females, white females, and black males) the corresponding frequencies were negligible (see Figure 3).

Roles and Stereotypes

Clark (1972), in analyzing the role of blacks in entertainment television, has observed that psychological legitimization of a group (or its aspirations) in the

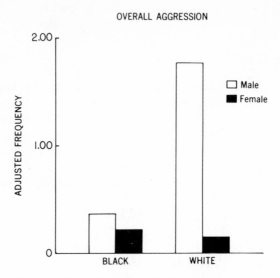

Figure 3. Mean frequency of aggressive acts per 5 minutes of screen appearance in nine racially mixed television programs. (Source: Donagher et al., 1975.)

entertainment medium involves two steps: recognition and respect. Certain groups may thus not be recognized, that is, they may be relegated to relative unimportance or even oblivion by television through being underrepresented or not even shown at all. The rare appearance of blacks on television during the 1950s, mostly in minor roles, serves as a clear example.

As legitimization progresses, recognition becomes less imbalanced and respect becomes an issue: Is the relevant group accorded dramatic roles (and behavioral repertoires within those roles) consistent with the real life roles and role relationships which it actually occupies or to which it aspires? Equally important, as Clark implies, recognition without respect may be as damaging as nonrecognition; *Amos and Andy* contributed to the stereotyping of blacks in a way *Playhouse 90* did not. A closer look at the data for the recognition and respect that various groups enjoy discloses an interesting if somewhat disconcerting picture.

Sex Roles

Few aspects of television play potentially greater importance for socialization than those involved in sex role portrayals; every program carries a lesson as to the differential expectations our society has for men and women.

Perhaps the most salient fact of all regarding sex roles on television is in terms of marked disparities in recognition. An early study (Head, 1954) disclosed that men held twice as many major roles on television as women. Perhaps as a concomitant of the increase in violent program themes, women actually enjoyed even less recognition in the 1960s; one analysis of 1967–1969 disclosed that women held only one-quarter of the major roles (Gerbner, 1972). Even on children's programs, males still outnumber females more than 2 to 1 (Sternglanz & Serbin, 1974).

In terms of respect, other differences appear: Only 20% of the TV roles having a definite occupational acitivity are held by women (DeFleur, 1964), with the "typical" female portrayal involving a romantic or sexual context (Gerbner, 1972). A closer look at respect, with particular reference to children's programs, has been reported by Sternglanz and Serbin (1974). In addition to confirming the well-established finding that TV females are substantially less aggressive than their male counterparts, these investigators reported that males tend to be rewarded more often than females for their behavior in televised roles. Men also are shown as significantly more planful and constructive, while women are portrayed as more deferent and more likely to be punished simply for emitting a high level of activity.

Ethnic and Racial Portrayals

Recognition and respect have been shown repeatedly to reflect unfavorably on ethnic and racial minorities in terms of their television portrayals. In an early study, Smythe (1954) found that 80% of all television characters were white Americans; of the remaining 20%, Europeans, especially of English and Italian extraction, appeared most frequently. Chinese characters accounted for only .2% of television's roles, despite the fact that more than one-fifth of the world's population is Chinese. Asian, Indian, and African characters, representing fully one-third of the world in real-life, were virtually unrepresented in American television. Roughly the same pattern has been in evidence for almost 20 years (Gerbner, 1972).

Turning to respect, for the same groups, we find that when minorities do achieve recognition through televised roles, they fare substantially less well than white Americans. Though the trend may have begun to change recently, for a long time the effective and powerful agent of law enforcement was almost invariably a white Anglo-American, while the inevitably vanquished villain was likely to be a central or southern European; Smythe (1954) reported that Italians were law breakers during more than half of their television appearances. And, again, the early pattern has continued. "Foreigners" wrote Gerbner (1972), "and those not identifiable as Americans [were in 1969] more likely to become involved in violence and more likely to pay a higher price for it than were the Americans" (p. 58).

Blacks, as we noted earlier, were almost unrecognized in the first years of television; their rare appearances were typically as small-time villains or lovable buffoons. Perhaps because black Americans have become a powerful, vocal, and relatively sophisticated self-interest group in the past 10 years, their television appearances have substantially increased in frequency and changed in role. Today blacks are likely to be presented as "regulators," staunch and law-abiding supporters of the middle-class status quo (Clark, 1972) who are nonviolent even as law enforcement officers and who, in the 1973–1974 season, tended to exhibit more prosocial behavior than their white counterparts (Donagher, Liebert, Poulos, & Davidson, 1974; see Figure 4).

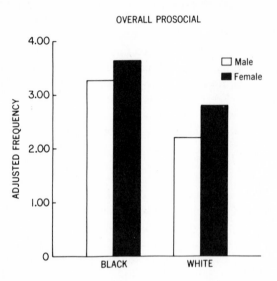

Figure 4.   Mean frequency of prosocial acts per 5 minutes of screen appearance in nine racially mixed television programs. (Source: Donagher et al., 1975.)

Occupational Roles and Social Class

Notwithstanding the intrepid Archie Bunker, blue collar workers are substantially underrepresented on television; fewer than one-tenth of all TV's entertainment characters are working class (Head, 1954; Gentile & Miller, 1961). The inevitable correlate of these facts is, of course, that professional workers and representatives of the middle and upper classes are overrepresented and thereby accorded undue recognition. DeFleur's (1964) analysis of occupational roles brings the point home. "While nearly half the males in the actual labor force," he wrote, "hold jobs in commerce and industry as operatives, craftsmen, and related workers, less than a tenth did so on television [where there were] more deep-sea divers than factory workers, more helicopter pilots than supermarket clerks, more nightclub singers than salesgirls" (pp. 68–72).

Respect for professional roles is generally high on television, but varies too much from occupation to occupation for many generalizations to be warranted. The prototypic television lawyer is clever and almost inevitably produces some unorthodox legal play; the usual artist cannot go half an hour without some temperamental outburst or display of eccentricity; private investigators are not only more charming but also far more capable than their police counterparts; and the underrepresented taxi, bus, and truck driver makes his occasional appearance as a burly, aggressive lout (DeFleur, 1964).

LEARNING AND COMPREHENSION: TELEVISION AS A TEACHER

"All television is educational television," former FCC Commissioner Nicholas Johnson once remarked. Research backs up Johnson's quip, showing that even programming designed primarily for entertainment conveys many lessons.

The first studies on the capacity of entertainment television to instruct, by teaching novel forms of physical and verbal aggression, are also the most widely known (e.g., Bandura, Ross, & Ross, 1961; 1963a; 1963b). These investigations showed that preschoolers would learn the component responses of complex motor sequences after exposure to a single animated television show. What is more, continuing the same line of demonstration, Hicks (1965) has shown that information extracted from a single exposure to simulated television content may be retained for periods of up to 6 months.

Acquisition of discrete physical acts and rote responses must nonetheless be distinguished from the learning and comprehension of deeper themes, norms, and relationships that televised content may convey. A growing body of evidence now warns us that young children may comprehend the content and meaning of televised materials—whether 30-second commercials or 2-hour dramatic specials—quite differently from adults, and thus leave the viewing situation with less, more, or even different information than would adults exposed to the same content. Young children for example, often will inaccurately interpret even "simple" underlying plots or perceive a program as a series of discrete and unrelated segments rather than as a continuing story; this is particularly true when the motives and consequences attending a character's actions are concerned (Collins, 1970; Leifer & Roberts, 1972).

The child's limited ability to comprehend and process all of television's nuances does not, of course, prevent socially relevant lessons from being learned; the youngster's simplistic interpretation and credulous perception of entertainment programming is as likely to enhance as to neutralize television's socializing influence. For example, interviewing 300 white elementary youngsters about equally representing urban, suburban, and rural schools, Greenberg (1972) reported that fully 40% said they had learned most about how blacks look, talk, and dress from television. In another study, DeFleur and

DeFleur (1967) interviewed and tested more than 200 children in the ages 6–13 about occupations with which they had minimal personal contact; there was far greater knowledge of the roles and status of those given high television exposure (e.g., judges, newspaper reporters, waiters, and bellhops) than those given low exposure (e.g., bank presidents, accountants, printers, and shipping clerks). What is more, high television users were more knowledgable than low-users about "television" occupations but did not differ from low users in their knowledge and evaluation of roles not often seen on television. Considering their data in aggregate, DeFleur and DeFleur concluded: " . . . within the present samples of children and occupations, television is a more potent source of occupational status knowledge than either personal contact or the general community culture" (1967, p. 787).

Recalling the frequency of stereotypic portrayals that have dominated the medium since the early 1950s, it is not surprising that high users of television and other pictorial media (i.e., movies and comic books) were found more likely to believe in and invoke social stereotypes than were low users, even after the possible effects of potentially confounding third variables (e.g., social class and IQ) were eliminated (Bailyn, 1959). Likewise, a pioneering experimental demonstration of the process (Siegel, 1958) contrasted the effects of two versions of a simulated radio play on second-grade children. The stories varied in that one presented taxicab drivers as aggressive, whereas the other did not. When questioned later, those who had heard the more aggressive story were more likely than controls to express the view that cab drivers in their own town were aggressive. Apparently, these youngsters had both acquired, accepted, and generalized the aspersion that was implicit in the program.

ACCEPTANCE OF THE TELEVISED MESSAGE

Findings described in the previous sections illustrate that television viewing is a major activity for children in the United States and throughout the world. What is more, the content seen is laced with behavioral examples of violence, and presents a view of groups, nations, and of life itself that is often disconcerting. From exposure to such content children learn specific responses that they may reproduce later, directly or in modified form; perhaps more important, they also acquire some of their first general impressions about society and their own place and that of others in it.

We now turn to a closer look at the remaining question dictated by our theoretical model, which is, perhaps, also the most important: To what degree do children exposed to television entertainment accept what they see as a guide for their own attitudes and actions?

The answer appears to be that such influences are often substantial, as evidenced by converging lines of research on several critical areas of socialization. By far the greatest documentation, however, is available for the acceptance of televised aggression.

The Impact of Televised Aggression

The first studies designed to explore the effects of televised aggression (e.g., many of the now classic "Bobo doll" studies) had great significance as demonstrations of a psychological process, but were waved aside by critics as being only tangentially relevant (or downright irrelevant) to human interpersonal aggression. In the decade following this early debate a vast amount of empirical evidence has been added to our store of knowledge, dramatically extending the earlier findings and substantially buttressing the validity of causal inferences drawn from them. Inasmuch as this work has been reviewed in detail elsewhere (e.g., Liebert, Davidson, & Neale, 1974) only a brief summary will be provided here.

Experimental Studies: Confirming the Causal Link

During the early 1970s, many experimental studies were reported that sought to confirm or disconfirm the hypothesized causal relationship between TV violence viewing and subsequent aggression. Preponderantly, they supported the conclusion that exposure to examples of aggressive behavior, directly taken from broadcast television, does increase aggressiveness in viewers through the entire age span from early childhood to late adolescence (e.g., Leifer & Roberts, 1972; Liebert & Baron, 1972; Steuer, Applefield, & Smith, 1971; Ellis & Sekyra, 1972; Stein & Friedrich, 1972). Ellis and Sekyra (1972), for example, showed first-grade children either an aggressive or neutral animated cartoon, taken directly from the program library of a local television station. The aggressive show featured hitting, tackling, kicking, and other typical forms of cartoon aggression; the neutral program was a musical variety show. Viewers exposed to the aggressive cartoon engaged in significantly more aggressive behavior when they returned to their classrooms than those who saw either the variety show or no television. What is perhaps most important about this study, and several others as well (e.g., Stein & Friedrich, 1972; Steuer et al., 1971), is that it demonstrates the direct effect of broadcast television as an instigator of overt physical aggression by one child against another.

In an extensive developmental study, Leifer and Roberts (1972) exposed 271 children (40 kindergarteners, 54 third, 56 sixth, 51 ninth, and 70 twelfth graders) to programs containing varying amounts of aggression. The shows were taken directly off the air without editing. After viewing, each child was questioned about his understanding of the motivations and consequences for the aggressive acts in each program and then asked to choose among various behavioral options in hypothetical conflict situations. After detailing other findings regarding comprehension of the televised material, the investigators state:

Finally, and most important, there was a significant main effect for amount of violence portrayed in the program, with the two most violent programs producing the most subsequent physical aggression and the two least violent programs producing the least subsequent physical aggression . . . [there was] no statistical support for the hypothesis that the effects of violent programming will change with the child's level of development . . . (pp. 87–89)

Correlational Field Studies

In addition to these experimental studies, and later ones as well (e.g., Drabman & Thomas, 1974), the link between exposure to television violence and acceptance of aggression as a mode of behavior is borne out by correlational studies. Here, the typical investigation involves determining the child's viewing habits (particularly his favorite programs or those watched most often) to obtain an estimate of exposure to aggressive television content; this information is then

Table 1.   Summary of Correlations Between Violence Viewing and Aggressiveness

Locale	Grade	N	Self-Report, Aggressive Behavior	Other-Report Aggressive Behavior
		Samples of boys		
New York	3	211	No data	+ +
Michigan	4–6	434	No data	+ +
Wisconsin	6–7	338	+	+
Maryland	7	122	+	0
Maryland	8–9	80	0	No data
Wisconsin	9–10	43	+	+ +
Maryland	10	107	+ +	+ +
		Samples of Girls		
New York	3	216	No data	0
Michigan	4–6	404	No data	+ + +
Wisconsin	6–7	30	+ +	+ +
Maryland	7	108	+ +	+ +
Wisconsin	9–10	40	+	+ +
Maryland	10	136	+	+

Source: Chaffee (1972), who notes: "Cell entries indicate presence of positive (+) or null (0) correlation between the amount of violence viewing reported by the adolescent, and an aggressiveness index based on the type of report listed in the column heading. Stronger or more consistent positive relationships are indicated by repeating the sign (+ +). These are very approximate estimates of the strength of the evidence that the correlation is non-zero" (p.25).

correlated with independently obtained information (peer reports, self-reports, public records) pertaining to each participant's approval and acceptance of aggression. The thrust of these findings, which have been thoughtfully reviewed by Chaffee (1972), is clear: For youngsters of both sexes and a variety of backgrounds and ages, television violence viewing is positively related to aggression as a mode of behavior. The overall pattern of results is captured well by Table 1.

Even more compelling than the pattern of synchronous correlations, there is a direct basis for concluding that aggressive television fare, as broadcast, can have a cumulative effect: Lefkowitz, Eron, Walder, and Huesmann's (1972) landmark time-lagged panel study, which spanned a ten-year period. In the late 1950s Lefkowitz and his associates correlated data from more than 400 nine-year-old youngsters on measures including peer ratings of aggression, self-reports of aggression, self-reports of various aspects of television viewing, and information on family background and parental practices; ten years later, when the participants were 19, similar measures were again correlated. Results disclosed that, for boys, exposure to television violence at age 9 was significantly linked to aggressive behavior ten years later at age 19. As seen in Figure 5, this effect was not limited to a small number of individuals who were already highly aggressive at age 9, but held for the entire spectrum of male adolescents (Huesmann, Eron, Lefkowitz, & Walder, 1973). Further statistical analyses of the path of this relationship disclosed that television violence had apparently *caused,* rather than merely been associated with, aggressive behavior (Kenny, 1972; Neale, 1972).

Social Stereotypes

From the point of view of an increasingly large number of social scientists, television entertainment has become a socializing force that shapes and cultivates the viewer's perceptions of the world. Perhaps no one has been better able to see the role of television in this broad light than George Gerbner, Dean of the Annenberg School of Communications. He has described the link between exposure and acceptance this way:

. . . television drama is in the mainstream—or is the mainstream—of the symbolic environment cultivating common conceptions of life, society, and the world . . . living deep in the mainstream, being a heavy consumer of its images and messages, mean more intensive acculturation and tighter integration of the myths and rituals of the symbolic world into one's view of how the real world works than does living a more insulated life or in a more independent or diversified cultural context. . . . more heavy viewers of television than light or nonviewers [should therefore] tend to conceive of reality as they experience it in the symbolic world of television drama. (Gerbner & Gross, 1974, p. 2.)

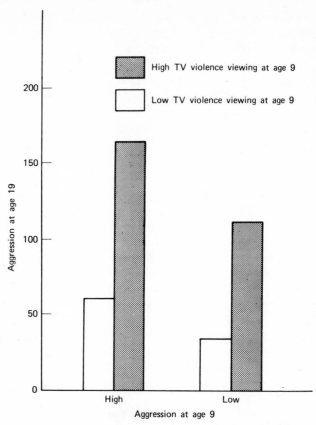

Figure 5.   Mean aggressive scores for boys at age 19 as a function of aggression at age 9 and television violence viewing at age 9, showing that high television violence viewing instigated later aggression regardless of initial level of aggression. (Source: Based on data reported in Huesmann, Eron, Lefkowitz, and Walder, 1973.)

Following this premise, Gerbner and his associates contrasted the perceptions of life held by a group of black junior high school youngsters, split into subsamples on the basis of whether they were heavy or light television viewers. The investigators devised a measure of cultural stereotypes by creating a set of 90 passport-type photographs of a heterogeneous group of people, taken under standard conditions, the characters being equally divided according to sex, race (black or white) and age (18–30 versus 35–60). As part of the research, heavy and light viewers were asked to sort through the photographs and identify (among other things) prospective heroes. Although all participants were black, heavy viewers were far more likely than light viewers to select white characters as heroes; they also were more likely to select male heroes. These differences appear to reflect a direct acceptance of the dramatic stereotypes of television into the heavy viewers' own perceptions of the world, including a disparaging of persons of their own race as being distinctly less heroic, and somewhat more villainous as well (Gerbner & Gross, 1974).

Parallel differences have been found for sex role stereotypes. Noting, as we have earlier in this chapter, that present fare shows men and women in very different ways, Frueh and McGhee (1974) reasoned that, if television inculcated this message, there would be a positive correlation between youngsters' overall exposure to television and the strength of their identification with the values stereotypically associated with their own gender (for example, girls' preferences for dolls, dishes, and dresses, and boys' perferences for trucks, guns, and tools). Specifically, they obtained detailed information about the viewing habits of a large number of children and identified 80 youngsters— 10 boys and 10 girls from kindergarten, second, fourth, and sixth grade—half of whom were high watchers (25 hours or more per week) and half of whom were low watchers (10 hours of less per week). Every participant was then administered the It Scale, a measure of sex role preference and identity that closely parallels the television stereotype. For every grade level, and for both sexes, high watchers showed significantly higher identification with the traditional sex role associated with their own gender than did low watchers.

The studies reviewed in this section are all correlational, and suffer from the weaknesses of that methodology. To our knowledge, experimental evidence of the impact of most televised social stereotypes has not yet been conducted, partly because of difficulties in conceptualizing appropriate treatment groups. Then too, acceptance of information bearing on one's identity and that of others is a gradual process, not readily susceptible to short-term change by variations of a program or two, as viewed in a laboratory setting. Effective experiments would seem to require a library of preanalyzed broadcast entertainment programs, making possible the creation of enriched diets of contrasting programs (e.g., shows featuring females in domestic or other "traditional" roles versus shows in which women characters enjoy social and professional status on a par with men). We shall return to this issue later.

ACCEPTANCE: PROSOCIAL EFFECTS

The possible effects of television extend into many spheres of socialization. Certainly, it is true that the greatest expenditure of effort among social scientists has focused on the transmission of aggression, social stereotypes, and other forms of behavior that may be troublesome to society. At the same time, though, researchers and broadcasters alike are becoming much more mindful of the positive effects which, incidentally or by design, television may foster.

In this section we shall describe some of these "prosocial effects" of television, as they have been disclosed by recent research.

Television as a Direct Educator: Cognitive Skills

By far, the best known effort to use network television as a transmitter of basic knowledge and cognitive skills is *Sesame Street* and its companion series, *The Electric Company,* both products of Children's Television Workshop. These series, first aired in 1969 and 1971, respectively, were specifically designed as distillates of effective educational curricula on the one hand (e.g., in teaching letter and number recognition, vocabulary, and, in the case of *Electric Company*, more advanced reading skills) and a snappy entertainment format on the other. Extensive reviews of CTW's efforts are now widely available (Lesser, 1974; Liebert et al., 1973), so a simple summary will suffice here. In studies done both in the United States (e.g., Ball & Bogatz, 1970; Bogatz & Ball, 1972) and abroad (e.g., Salomon, 1974) *Sesame Street* has been shown to successfully capture and hold child audiences in direct competition with commercial entertainment programming; at the same time, it is a remarkably effective teacher for both middle-class and disadvantaged children. What is more, a followup study of children who had been heavy or light viewers during their preschool years revealed that, on entering school, heavy viewers were better prepared than light viewers; those who had viewed frequently also continued to outgain low viewers and to score significantly higher on measures of attitudes toward school and toward people of races other than their own as well (Bogatz & Ball, 1972).

CTW's work was designed as an experimental prototype—a demonstration of what other broadcasters might do—and not merely as a "one-shop" corner on the market (Lesser, 1974). Slowly, but inevitably, the pioneers have begun to be imitated. Henderson, Zimmerman, Swanson, and Bergan (1974), for example, have begun work on programming specifically aimed at providing cognitive skill instruction for American Indian children.

Relying heavily on basic theory and research on observational learning and systematic formative research, Henderson and his associates produced a series of short programs designed to teach such complex skills as conservation, seriation, and the ability to form effective questions; at the same time, the programs were specifically designed to be culturally relevant for the Papago Indian children for whom they were made. For example, the program backgrounds were set in an artistic representation of a desert environment and the human characters were Papago women who spoke in both English and native Papago; the principal "props" were baskets, saguaro ribs, cholla branches, and hand puppets representing Papago children; the background music was specifically selected for its similarity to the tribe's traditional music. At the same time, of course, the investigators also capitalized on more universal principles now known to maximize television's impact. Each scene was kept short (that is, between 2 and 3 minutes), characters and visual background material were varied from scene to scene, and when sedentary segments were required for pedagogic purposes, they were alternated with supportive action sequences to maintain a varied and interesting pace. Music and song were used not only to maintain interest; the lyrics were also part of the instructional package, as illustrated by "The Question Song" (See Table 2).

Table 2.   "The Question Song" Used in the Television Programs of Henderson et al., Illustrating the Use of Musical Lyrics for Instructional Purposes.

If you see something that is not clear
Think of a question and find someone to hear
If with a question you always start
Everyone will think you are very smart.

Oh, Why is the flower upside down?
How come her head is next to the ground?
What would happen if she were to fall?
It would be much better if she stood tall.

There are lots of people who know a lot.
They know many things that we do not
We can ask them questions and find out too
And with all the answers we'll be smart too!

Continually revising their programs in response to data collected at each step, the investigators succeeded quite unambiguously in producing the desired results. As observed in their first-year report,

The magnitude of significant effects increased systematically from the second to the last study. Not only were the results of the seriation and question-asking studies unambiguous and highly significant, but the outcomes were also of clear practical significance. The absolute magnitude of mean change attributable to the experimental treatment was impressive, but perhaps as important was the fact that gains were made by a very high percentage of the children. . . . In the last two experiments of the first year's work on this project, practically every child made gains which could reasonably be attributed to the television instruction. (p. 59.)

Interpersonal Prosocial Behavior

As far back as the early 1960s, investigators began to explore the possible ability of television formats to transmit various forms of prosocial behavior to children. Employing brief, simulated television programs, it was soon demonstrated that the medium could be used to transmit a wide gamut of behaviors including sharing (Bryan, 1970; Bryan & Walbek, 1970a, 1970b; Elliot & Vasta 1971), rule adherence (Stein & Bryan, 1972; Wolf & Cheyne, 1972), delay of gratification (Yates, 1974), increased social interaction with peers (O'Connor, 1969), and affection (Fryrear & Thelen, 1969).

Thus far, however, there have been remarkably few demonstrations of the effects of braodcast television on prosocial behavior. A notable exception was the pioneering demonstration of Stein and Friedrich (1972; Friedrich & Stein, 1973) who exposed approximately 100 preschool boys and girls to one of three 12-program diets: aggressive (*Batman* and *Superman* cartoons), neutral (shows featuring such activities as children working on a farm), and prosocial (episodes from the series *Misterogers' Neighborhood*). Before the viewing period, during its course and for 2 weeks thereafter, each youngster's behavior was recorded unobtrusively in the naturalistic nursery school situation by trained observers who were blind to the particular diets of the children whose behavior they watched. In the category of *self-control* (which included rule obedience, tolerance of delay, and task persistence—all emphasized in the *Misterogers* series), children exposed to the prosocial programming generally increased (and those exposed to the aggressive diet decreased) relative to those who saw neutral shows. Likewise, interpersonal prosocial behaviors (e.g., cooperation, nurturance toward others, verbalizing one's own feelings) also tended to increase as a result of the prosocial programming for those who had come from the lower half of the socioeconomic range.

As a direct demonstration of what broadcast television can do, the work of Stein and Friedrich represents a giant step. Nonetheless, the investigation was limited by the presence of a number of uncontrolled factors that somewhat restrict both its theoretical and practical significance. Among these are wide variations in the program format among the three diets, appreciable differences in the type of characters displayed, and quite different mixes in the relative balance of entertainment and instructional components. What is more, *Misterogers* is not a competitive network program, and its exhortative, often sedentary format might well limit the size of its audience.

For these reasons a study in our laboratory (Sprafkin, Liebert, & Poulos, 1975) was designed to determine whether the presence of a particular prosocial act (in this case, helping), appearing in a highly successful commercial show, would increase the occurrence of similar behavior in young viewers. To control for the basic format attributes, we selected for our principal treatments two programs from the *Lassie* series. Both shows featured the same major human and canine characters, took place in the same setting, were written for the same general audience, and presumably were motivated by the same entertainment and commercial interests. Though other differences in story line were necessarily present, from our perspective the critical difference between the episodes was that one of them had a specific altruistic example by a child character woven into it while the other did not. We reasoned that the combination of controlled similarity in format dimensions and a "naturally occurring" variation of socially relevant content provided the ideal circumstance to focus on the potential effect of specific modeling cues from completely unedited entertainment television. As a further control, a third group of children were shown an episode from the pleasant *Brady Bunch* series.

Inasmuch as the prosocial example in the *Lassie* episode showed Jeff (the central child character) risk his life by hanging over the ledge of a mine shaft to save a puppy, we created a behavioral test situation—designed to appear unrelated to the seemingly fortuitous television viewing experience that preceded it—in which our subjects (first-grade boys and girls) had to choose between earning prizes on a special game or helping puppies themselves, albeit without risk of life or limb.

Results showed clearly that the basic hypothesis was confirmed. Exposure to the prosocial *Lassie* show produced significantly more helping than either of the control programs, which did not differ from one another (see Figure 6).

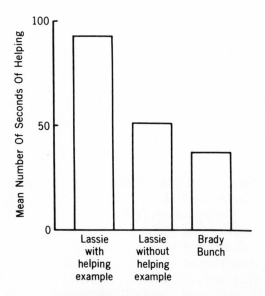

Figure 6. Mean number of seconds of helping by children who had viewed the prosocial *Lassie,* neutral *Lassie,* and *Brady Bunch* program. (Source: Sprafkin, Liebert, and Poulos, 1975.)

REFINING THE INQUIRY: NEW DIRECTIONS IN RESEARCH

While material reviewed in previous sections leaves little doubt that television does act as a socializing force—and a powerful one—for young viewers, another fact is equally clear: Our knowledge of the specific effects and precise psychological mechanisms involved is still very limited. In our own laboratory we have been concerned, over the past two years, with the task of developing improved procedures and more sophisticated methodologies that can be brought to bear on the study of television's impact. In the present section we will describe two of these efforts, and also use the occasion to introduce some new findings they have yielded.

Creating Adequate "Television Diets" for Research

In naturalistic correlational studies of the effects of television, information about the content to which a child has been exposed is usually obtained from the subject himself. Often this simply involves the gross measure of overall amount of television use (e.g., to form groups of "heavy" and "light" users). But the child who watches 30 hours of *Sesame Street, Zoom, Misterogers Neighborhood,* and *The Waltons* every week is exposed to very different lessons than the child who views 30 hours of *Mannix, Mod Squad,* and *Spiderman;* when both children are simply classified as "heavy viewers" valuable information about exposure is obscured and the power of research is markedly reduced.

A somewhat more effective procedure involves obtaining information as to the *particular* programs which the child regularly views and then rating these to provide an assessment of the child's putative, self-imposed diet of socially relevant examples. This has been done by requesting participants to list their favorite programs, or the programs they watch most often; some investigators have taken the additional step of asking children (or, for younger participants, their parents) to keep a diary of television viewing for a period of a week or more.

Even here, though, rough and ready guesses by the investigators as to which programs are the most violent (or the most prosocial) may represent program stereotypes at least as much as they reflect the actual content of the programs themselves, a problem compounded by the fact that programs within a series may vary widely in terms of the amount of socially relevant examples which they contain. (In our own work, we have found series in which one program was quite prosocial and almost devoid of aggressive examples, while another show from the same series was highly aggressive and had little prosocial content.) Clearly, a general rating of such a series would provide less than ideal information about the kind of input received by viewers. This is not to say, of course, that estimates of degree of exposure to a given content in such correlational studies are useless; they do partially reflect the desired information, but contain measurement error as well.

In experimental studies, however, imprecision is unnecessary. Procedures can be devised for coding the presence of any type of socially relevant information and, if such analyses are performed on a sufficiently large and diverse amount of programming, contrasting "diets" suitable to testing almost any hypothesis can be created and their effects determined through controlled research.

We have been developing just such a procedure. Our aim is to produce a large pool of programming with every program described and coded according to its socially relevant content. From this pool, we reasoned, investigators in our own laboratory and elsewhere would be able to draw substantial "diets" tailor-made to serve almost any experimental hypothesis while maximizing control on as many theoretically irrelevant factors as possible.

The first step was to develop a coding system that would reliably differentiate and identify categories of potential interest. The formative work was spearheaded by Emily S. Davidson and John M. Neale, who have described the system in detail elsewhere (Davidson and Neale, 1974). The code that finally emerged contains eight categories, listed and defined in Table 3.

As the table makes clear, the categories represent many of the behaviors of traditional concern to workers interested in socialization, including self-control, interpersonal prosocial behavior, and, of course, aggression. On the other hand, as Davidson and Neale have detailed, pragmatic considerations (such as limitations in the televised material itself) served to define and limit the scope of this effort.

We have now coded over 300 programs according to each of the categories and obtained supplemental information about race, sex, and age of principal characters and plot summaries as well. Research using the diet pool is just beginning but examination of its contents, representing a wide range of shows, reveals some fascinating information. First of all, there is an impressive availability of prosocial examples in contemporary television in the category of altruism and a considerable amount of sympathy. Interestingly, though, there is little resistance to temptation and, despite the high level of aggression, almost no control of aggressive impulses. It is clear, then, that television exposes its viewers to strong doses of some social behaviors to the virtual exclusion of others (see Table 3). It would be a mistake, of course, automatically to assume that learning and acceptance of these examples are equal across the categories, but we are now in the position to test this hypothesis and innumerable others by controlling input far better than we previously could.

As a first attempt to use the pool for creating experimental diets, we have sorted the shows into broad aggressive, neutral, and prosocial types. (Approximately 20% of the pool did not fit our criteria for any of these categories.) Table 4 describes the content of the diets that emerged. In collaboration with Paul Ekman and Randall Harrison, we will be determining their effects in a

Table 3. Mean Number of Socially Relevant Examples per Program Hour in 309 Programs Broadcast on Network and Independent Stations Between May 28, 1974 and August 21, 1974, with a Brief Definition of Each Category

Category	Mean Frequency per Hour
Altruism Acts of sharing, helping and cooperation	11.15
Aggression Acts involving the use of force, threat of force, or intent of force against another person or animal	7.28
Sympathy Verbal or behavioral expressions of concern for others or their problems	5.95
Explaining feelings of self or others Statements to another person explaining the feelings, thinking, or action of others with the intent of effecting positive outcome, including increasing the understanding of others, resolving strife, smoothing out difficulties, or reassuring someone	3.16
Reparation for bad behavior Behavior that is clearly intended as reparation for an act seen as wrongdoing committed by the person himself	2.21
Delay of gratification/task persistence Postponing a small reward for a larger one and/or spending additional time or effort on a task so that a goal may be reached or a product made better	1.94
Resistance to temptation Withstanding the temptation to engage in behaviors generally prohibited by society (e.g., stealing)	.61
Control of aggressive impulses Nonaggressive acts or statements that serve to eliminate or prevent aggression by self or others	.49

Table 4. Mean Number of Socially Relevant Examples in Major Categories per Program Hour for the Aggressive, Neutral, and Prosocial Diets Developed for Naturalistic Research

	Aggressive	Neutral	Prosocial
Altruism	6.02	9.56	16.50
Aggression	26.86	.52	.58
Sympathy	4.64	4.16	8.80
Explaining feeling of self or others	1.66	2.58	4.84
Reparation for bad behavior	1.10	2.00	3.22
Delay of gratification/task persistence	1.28	1.30	3.10

field experimental study to be conducted in Micronesia, where television has not yet been introduced to most of the islands. A number of smaller-scale field experimental investigations, focusing on individual types of televised social example, also will be underway shortly.

Direct Applications: Contributing to Television Production

There is substantial need to translate the work of the researcher into usable information for those developing children's programs. In this last section we describe one such effort, a collaborative project devoted to the production of 30-second spots (the length of most commercials) to teach cooperative behavior through observational learning.

The project began when the communications branch of a large Protestant denomination, the United Methodist Church, approached us with the question: What positive steps can be taken to improve children's television? After much discussion, it became clear that production of actual television fare for broadcast use was ideal. Here we could involve the research team in a product that would be seen on the commercial airwaves; success, if our understanding of children and television could lead us to it, would carry with it a visible and palpable demonstration that prosocial television could work, and that the researcher did indeed have something useful to say to the broadcaster.

Following our own theory and research as far as possible, we envisioned each spot as presenting an interpersonal conflict that could—but does not—result in aggression and/or violence. Instead, the television peer models were to act in a cooperative way that led to a solution satisfactory to all parties. This theme, that troublesome interactions can be satisfactorily settled by positive means, was chosen because it represents a situation that arises often in most children's (and adult's) lives.

Major Principles and Their Translation

In designing and testing these short messages, we drew on many concepts. A few of them, however, can be singled out as particularly central.

1. Present the same basic theme in more than one spot. Much basic research on observational learning suggests that even quite young children can abstract underlying principles from the behavior of others, and then apply these principles in new and diverse situations (e.g., Liebert & Swenson, 1971; Zimmerman & Rosenthal, 1974). Thus, the successful practice of cooperation was to be presented in three stories, varying across situations, settings, and models. In this way, generalization was built in rather than merely hoped for.

2. Choose situations that will optimize immediate recognition and understanding by child viewers. It has been shown that new information is most likely to be understood and accepted if it is contacted in an already familiar situation. Such presentations are likely to optimally capture and hold attention and are likely to facilitate learning (Lesser, 1970).

3. *Emphasize physical action.*   Initial findings from our laboratory and that of others indicate that action is important for children's attention. For exposure as brief as 30 seconds, it might be particularly critical to capture attention in the beginning of the sequence.

4. *Use verbal statements to complement action and explicate both the conflict and solution.*   Labeling the positive behavior to which viewers are being exposed has been shown repeatedly to facilitate both learning and generalization of the lesson (e.g., Liebert & Allen, 1967; Liebert, Hanratty, & Hill, 1969).

5. *Accentuate the positive consequences of the modeled behavior.*   An enormous number of experiments have now shown that acceptance of a model's behavior is greatly facilitated when his/her outcomes are shown to be positive, that is, when vicarious reward is part of the observational learning experience. We have discussed this issue extensively elsewhere (Liebert & Poulos, 1973).

6. *Within each story, present two or more characters behaving in the desired way.*   Such presentations, involving multiple rather than single modeling, have been shown repeatedly to enhance the acceptance of the exemplary class of behavior (e.g., Bandura, Grusec, & Menlove, 1967; Liebert & Fernandez, 1970; McMains & Liebert, 1968).

Testing the Spots: Strategy

Evaluation of children's reactions to television programs designed for them has been the exception rather than the rule. (Series pilots, which yield a measure of a program's appeal before a large commitment is made, are often aired for adult shows, but rarely for children's [Liebert, Neale, & Davidson, 1973].) Testing, of course, lies at the heart of our work.

More specifically, our research effort involves three separate prongs, following directly from our theoretical model of observational learning. We evaluate the spots for the attraction they hold for youngsters (exposure), the clarity with which they convey the intended message (acquisition), and overt changes they produce in attitudes or behavior (acceptance). Within this framework our strategy involves testing each promising spot idea in a rough film version and altering it according to the results of this first, formative research; then we retest to see if the alterations have been effective; a final version is produced only after all test results are satisfactory. The success of this strategy can be illustrated by describing the final round of research on *The Swing,* a spot that was first aired on network television in May, 1974, and has since appeared on all three major networks and numerous independent stations.

The Swing opens with a boy and girl, approximately 8 to 10 years of age, running across a field to reach a swing on a playground and beginning to struggle over it, each claiming first rights. After a moment during which battle seems inevitable, one of the youngsters produces the insight that they should take turns and, significantly for the example, suggests that the other child go first. The last seconds show each of the children taking her or his turn, joyfully swinging through the air with the help of the other. In the background an adult is pushing a youngster on another swing, providing a slightly different example of positive social behavior. Figure 7 shows scenes from *The Swing*.

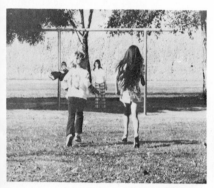
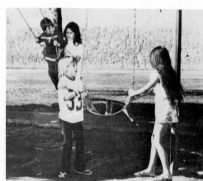
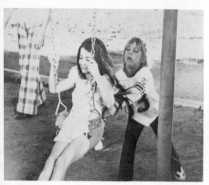
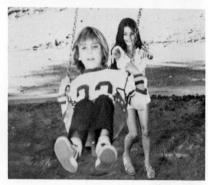

Figure 7. Scenes from *The Swing* depicting conflict and the satisfactory outcome of a cooperative resolution.

Exposure: Self-Controlled Attention

To provide a final evaluation of *The Swing's* power to hold attention, 4- to 9-year-old boys and girls (our target audience) were invited to watch regular television entertainment programming. The material viewed was altered slightly so as to be interrupted by *The Swing* and commercial spots that we had selected. To control for possible artifacts, half of the children watched one show and half another; the location of *The Swing* within each also was systematically rotated.

While the children watched television, a concealed videotape camera was used to monitor and record their faces, and this information was multiplexed with the material the children actually watched to produce a split-screen recording (see Figure 8). Thereafter, pairs of trained observers separately but simultaneously rated the amount of attention that each child gave to any bit of programming, as shown on the video record. These data allowed us to make a direct comparison of *The Swing* with two other spots for product commercials (see Figure 9). Note that *The Swing* more effectively captured the attention of the full range of children for whom it was intended; it is not simply that the other two spots were watched less (although on the average the were) but rather that—probably unknown to their creators—the other spots successfully reached only a subgroup of their intended audience. The prosocial *Swing*,

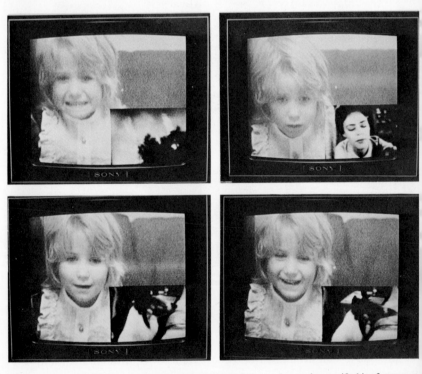

Figure 8.   A split screen recording that reveals the child's reaction to the specific bit of programming (lower right) he was viewing at that moment.

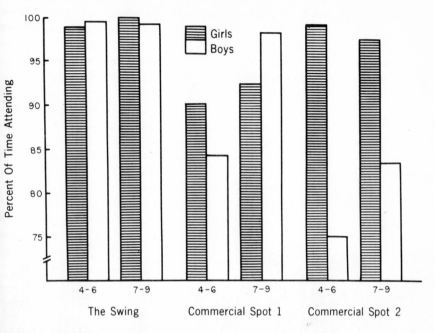

Figure 9. Mean percentage of time children of 4–6 and 7–9 years attended to *The Swing* and two product commercials.

in contrast, not only did not turn children away but appeared to interest them uniformly when presented in the way in which it eventually will appear on broadcast television, against the background of entertainment shows and product commercials.

Acquisition

The purpose of evaluating acquisition simply is to ascertain that children do indeed understand the lesson being presented. Our measure consisted of showing *The Swing* on a television monitor to 4- to 9-year-old children and interviewing them about its content. It was necessary from our point of view that the specific setting of the spot, as well as the primary message, be understood. Youngsters thus were asked to cite the most important thing about the story, the location and activity depicted, the actual conflict, and the resolution of the problem. Overall comprehension averaged 93% with a range of 85–100% for the various questions.

It is interesting to note that although the purpose of the acquisition measure seems obvious, its value is particularly evident when understanding is low. Comprehension tests of initial productions of alternative spots revealed that, on the average, only 38–67% of the questions asked were acceptably answered. (Judged inadequate in this regard, these spots were revised). A test of one regularly broadcast children's commercial that, like the spots, contains a brief story line, also showed 67% comprehension. These results, some of which are shown in Figure 10, provide striking evidence for the need for adequate evaluation of understanding by youngsters of even the very short messages they are presented on television.

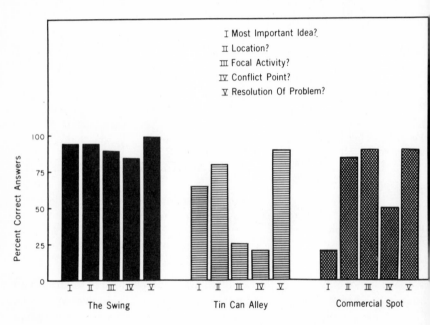

Figure 10. Mean percentage of correct answers to questions (I–V) about the content of *The Swing,* a potential alternative spot (*Tin Can Alley*), and a product commercial.

Acceptance

To evaluate the effects of *The Swing* on behavior, boys and girls from the second and fourth grades of a public school were given the opportunity to view twice consecutively either *The Swing* or one of two children's commercials. They then played a game in which they could earn points in order to win a prize; the larger the number of points, the better the prize. The game was designed so that cooperation could facilitate both children earning points. The choice was thus to cooperate for mutual benefit or "fight it out" to assure one's own positive outcome, a choice not unlike the one faced by the exemplars in *The Swing*.

The mean number of seconds of cooperation and competition was calculated

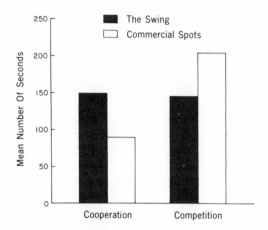

Figure 11. Mean number of seconds children cooperated and competed after viewing *The Swing* or product commercials.

for children who saw *The Swing* and for those who saw the commercials. *The Swing* group cooperated for an average of 151 seconds and competed for an average of 146 seconds; youngsters who had viewed commercials cooperated for 89 seconds and competed for 207 seconds, on the average. Watching *The Swing* clearly made cooperation a more likely outcome (See Figure 11).

A FINAL COMMENT

The work described above is doubtless recognizable as a progress report rather than a definitive statement and, in fact, that is the status of all the work to date on television as a shaper of personality. One thing, though, is clear: this entertainment medium is having a substantial and complex impact on children. The impact is present whether it is planned and understood or unplanned and overlooked. To us it seems clear which of these is the better path.

REFERENCES

Bailyn, L. Mass media and children: A study of exposure habits and cognitive effects. *Psychology Monographs,* 1959, **73,** 1, Whole No. 471.

Ball, S. & Bogatz, G. A. *The first year of Sesame Street: An evaluation.* Princeton, N.J.: Educational Testing Service, 1970.

Bandura. A., Grusec, J. E., & Menlove, F. L. Vicarious extinction of avoidance behavior. *Journal of Personality and Social Psychology,* 1967, **5,** 16–23.

Bandura, A. & Harris, M. B. Modification of syntactic style. *Journal of Experimental Child Psychology,* 1967, **4,** 341–352.

Bandura, A., Ross, D., & Ross, S. Imitation of film-mediated aggressive models. *Journal of Abnormal and Social Psychology,* 1963, **66,** 3–11. (a)

Bandura, A., Ross D., & Ross, S. Vicarious reinforcement and imitative learning. *Journal of Abnormal and Social Psychology,* 1963, **67,** 601–607. (b)

Bandura, A., & Ross, S.A. Transmission of aggression through imitation of aggressive models. *Journal of Abnormal and Social Psychology,* 1961, **63,** 575–582.

Bogatz, G. A. & Ball, S. *The second year of Sesame Street: A continuing evaluation.* Princeton, N.J.: Educational Testing Service, 1972.

Bogart, L. Warning: The Surgeon General has determined that TV violence is moderately dangerous to your child's mental health. *Public Opinion Quarterly,* 1972, **36,** 491–521.

Bryan, J. H. Children's reactions to helpers: Their money isn't where their mouths are. In J. Macauley & L. Berkowitz (Eds.), *Altruism and helping behavior.* New York: Academic Press, 1970.

Bryan, J. H. & London, P. Altruistic behavior by children. *Psychological Bulletin,* 1970, **73,** 200–211.

Bryan, J. H. & Walbek, N. H. Preaching and practicing generosity: Children's actions and reactions. *Child Development,* 1970, **41,** 329–353. (a)

Bryan, J. H. & Walbek, N. H. The impact of words, deeds and power upon children's altruistic behavior. *Child Development,* 1970, **41,** 747–757. (b)

Chaffee, S. H. Television and adolescent aggressiveness (overview). In G. A. Comstock & E. A. Rubinstein (Eds.), *Televison and social behavior. Vol. III: Television and adolescent aggressiveness.* Washington, D.C.: U.S. Government Printing Office, 1972, pp. 1–34.

Clark, C. Race, identification, and television violence. In G. A. Comstock, E. A. Rubinstein, & J. P. Murray (Eds.). *Television and social behavior. Vol. V: Television's effects: Further explorations.* Washington, D. C.: U.S. Government Printing Office, 1972, pp. 120–184.

Collins, W. A. Learning of media content: A developmental study. *Child Development,* 1970, **41,** 1133–1142.

Dahlgren, P. Television in the socialization process: Structures and programming of the Swedish Broadcasting Corporation. In G. A. Comstock & E. A. Rubinstein (Eds.). *Television and social behavior. Vol. I: Media content and control.* Washington, D. C.: U.S. Government Printing Office, 1972, pp. 533–546.

Davidson, E. S. & Neale, J. M. Analyzing prosocial content on entertainment television. Paper presented at the 82nd Annual Convention of the American Psychological Association, September 1, 1974; New Orleans.

DeFleur, M. Occupational roles as portrayed on television. *Public Opinion Quarterly,* 1964, **28,** 57–74.

DeFleur, M. L. & DeFleur, L. The relative contribution of television as a learning source for children's occupational knowledge. *American Sociological Review,* 1967, **32,** 777–789.

DeFleur, M. L. *Theories of mass communication.* New York: McKay, 1970.

Dominick, J. R. & Greenberg, B. S. Attitudes toward violence: The interaction of television exposure, family attitudes, and social class. In G. A. Comstock & E. A. Rubinstein (Eds.). *Television and social behavior. Vol. III: Television and adolescent aggressiveness.* Washington D. C.: U.S. Government Printing Office, 1972, pp. 314–335.

Donagher, P., Poulos, R. W., Liebert, R. M., & Davidson, E. S. Race, sex and social example: An analysis of inter-racial television entertainment. Unpublished manuscript, Media Action Research Center and State University of New York at Stony Brook, 1975.

Drabman, R. S. & Thomas, M. H. Does media violence increase children's toleration of real life aggression? *Developmental Psychology,* 1974, 10, 418–421.

Elliott, R., & Vasta, R. The modeling of sharing: Effects associated with vicarious reinforcement, symbolization, age, and generalization. *Journal of Experimental Child Psychology,* 1970, **10,** 8–15.

Ellis, G. T. & Sekyra, F. The effect of aggressive cartoons on the behavior of first grade children. *Journal of Psychology,* 1972, **81,** 37–43.

Friedrich, L. K., & Stein, A. H. Aggressive and prosocial television programs and the natural behavior of preschool children. *Society for Research in Child Development,* 1973, **38** (whole Monogr.).

Frueh, T., & McGhee, P. E. Traditional sex-role development and amount of time spent watching television. *Developmental Psychology,* 1975, 11, 109.

Fryrear, J. L., & Thelen, M. H. Effect of sex of model and sex of observer on the imitation of affectionate behavior. *Developmental Psychology,* 1969, **1,** 298.

Gardner. L. W. A content analysis of Japanese and American television. *Journal of Broadcasting,* 1961, **6,** 54–52.

Gentile, F. & Miller, S. M. Television and social class. *Sociology and Social Research,* 1961, **45,** 259–264.

Gerbner, G. Statement before the subcommittee on communications, United States Senate. In *Violence on Television: Hearings before the Subcommittee on Communications of the Committee on Commerce, Ninety-third Congress, Second Session.* 1974, Serial No. 93–76, pp. 56–105.

Gerbner, G. Violence in television drama: Trends and symbolic functions. In G. A. Comstock & A. E. Rubinstein (Eds.); *Television and social behavior. Vol I: Media content and control.* Washington, D. C.: U.S. Government Printing Office, 1972, pp. 28–187.

Gerbner, G., & Gross, L. Cultural indicators: The social reality of television drama. Unpublished manuscript. The Annenberg School of Communications, University of Pennsylvania, 1974.

Greenberg, B. S. Children's reactions to TV blacks. *Journalism Quarterly,* 1972, **49,** 5–14.

Halloran, J. D. & Croll, P. Television programs in Great Britian: Content and control (a pilot study). In G. A. Comstock and E. A. Rubinstein (Eds.); *Television and social behavior. Vol I: Media content and control.* Washington, D. C.: U.S. Government Printing Office, 1972, pp. 415–492.

Hapkiewicz, W. G. & Roden, A. H. The effects of aggressive cartoons on children's interpersonal play. *Child Development,* 1971, **42,** 1583–1585.

Henderson, R.W., Zimmerman, B. J., Swanson, R., & Bergan, J. R. Televised cognitive skill instruction for Papago native American children. Tucson, Arizona: Arizona Center for Educational Research and Development, 1974.

Head, S. Content analysis of television drama programs. *Film Quarterly,* 1954, **9,** 175–194.

Hicks, D. J. Imitation and retention of film-mediated aggressive peer and adult models. *Journal of Personality and Social Psychology,* 1965, **2,** 95–100.

Huesmann, L. R., Eron, L. D., Lefkowitz, M. M., & Walder, L. O. Television violence and aggression: The causal effect remains. *American Psychologist,* 1973, **28,** 617–620.

Johnson, N. *How to talk back to your television set.* Boston: Atlantic-Little, Brown and Company, 1967.

Kenny, D. A. Threats to the internal validity of cross-lagged panel inference, as related to "Television violence and child aggression: A followup study." In G. A. Comstock and E. A. Rubinstein (Eds.). *Television and social behavior Vol. III: Television and adolescent aggressiveness.* Washington, D.C.: U.S. Government Printing Office, 1972, pp. 136–140.

Lefkowitz, M. M., Eron, L. D., Walder, L. O., & Husemann, L. R. Television violence and child aggression: A followup study. In G. A. Comstock and E. A. Rubinstein (Eds.), *Television and social behavior. Vol. III: Television and adolescent aggressiveness.* Washington, D.C.: U. S. Government Printing Office, 1972, pp. 35–135.

Leifer, A. & Roberts, D. Children's responses to television violence. In J. P. Murray, E. A. Rubinstein, & G. A. Comstock (Eds.); *Television and social behavior. Vol. II: Television and social learning.* Washington, D.C.: U.S. Government Printing Office, 1972, pp. 43–180.

Lesser, G. S. *Children and television: Lessons from Sesame Street.* New York: Random House, 1974.

Lesser, G. S. Designing a program for broadcast television. In F. F. Korten, S. W. Cook, & J. I. Lacey (Eds.), *Psychology and the problems of society.* Washington, D.C.: American Psychology Association, 1970.

Liebert, R. M. Observational learning: Some social applications. In P. J. Elich (Ed.), *Fourth western symposium on learning.* Bellingham, Washington: Western Washington State College, 1973.

Liebert, R. M. Television and social learning: Some relationships between viewing violence and behaving aggressively (overview). In J. P. Murray, E. A. Rubinstein, & G. A. Comstock (Eds.), *Television and social behavior. Vol. II: Television and social learning.* Washington, D. C.: U. S. Government Printing Office, 1972, pp. 1–42.

Liebert, R. M. & Allen, M. K. The effects of rule structure and reward magnitude on the acquisition and adoption of self-reward criteria. *Psychological Reports,* 1967, **21**, 445–452.

Liebert, R. M. & Baron, R. A. Some immediate effects of televised violence on children's behavior. *Developmental Psychology,* 1972, **6**, 469–475.

Liebert, R. M. & Fernandez, L. E. Effects of single and multiple modeling cues on establishing norms for sharing. *Proceedings of the 78th Annual convention of the American Psychological Association,* 1970, pp. 437–438.

Liebert, R. M., Neale, J. M., & Davidson, E. S. *The early window: Effects of television on children and youth.* New York: Pergamon Press, 1973.

Liebert, R. M., Hanratty, M., & Hill, J. A. Effects of rule structure and training method on the adoption of a self-imposed standard. *Child Development,* 1969, **40**, 93–101.

Liebert, R. M., Odom, R. D., Hill, J. H., & Huff, R. Effects of age and rule familiarity on the production of modeled language constructions. *Developmental Psychology,* 1969, **1**, 108–112.

Liebert, R. M., & Poulos, R. W. Vicarious consequences as a source of information: a reply to Peed and Forehand. *Journal of Experimental Child Psyhcology,* 1973, **16**, 534–541.

Liebert, R. M., & Swenson, S. A. Abstraction, inference, and the process of imitative learning. *Developmental Psychology, 1971, 5, 500–504.*

Lyle, J. & Hoffman, H. R. Children's use of television and other media. In E. A. Rubinstein, G. A. Comstock, & J. P. Murray (Eds.), *Television and social behavior. Vol. IV: Television in day-to-day life: Patterns of use.* Washington, D.C.: U.S. Government Printing Office, 1972, pp. 129–256.

Maccoby, E. Effects of the mass media. In M. Hoffman & L. Hoffman (Eds.), *Review of child development research. Vol. I.* New York: Russell Sage Foundation, 1964.

McIntyre, J. J. & Teevan, J. J., Jr. Television violence and deviant behavior. In G. A. Comstock and E. A. Rubinstein (Eds.), *Television and social behavior. Vol. III: Television and adolescent aggressiveness.* Washington, D.C.: U.S. Government Printing Office, 1972, pp. 383–435.

McMains, M. J., & Liebert, R. M. The effects of discrepancies between successively modeled self-reward criteria on the adoption of a self-imposed standard, *Journal of Personality and Social Psychology,* 1968, **8**, 166–171.

Neale, J.M. Comment on "Television violence and child aggression: A followup study." In G. A. Comstock and E. A. Rubinstein (Eds.), *Television and social behavior. Vol. III: Television and adolescent aggressiveness.* Washington, D.C.: U.S. Government Printing Office, 1972, pp. 141–148.

O'Connor, R. D. Modification of social withdrawal through symbolic modeling. *Journal of Applied Behavior Analysis,* 1969, **2,** 15–22.

Peterson, R. C., Thurstone, L. L., Shuttleworth, F. K., & May, M. A. *Motion pictures and the social attitudes of children.* New York: The MacMillan Co., 1933.

Preston, M. I. Children's reactions to movie horrors and radio crime. *Journal of Pediatrics,* 1941, **19,** 147–168.

Robinson, J. P. Television's impact on everyday life: Some cross-national evidence. In E. A. Rubinstein, G. A. Comstock, & J. P. Murray (Eds.), *Television and social behavior. Vol. IV: Television in day-to-day life: Patterns of use.* Washington, D. C.: U.S. Government Printing Office, 1972, pp. 410–431.

Rosenhan, D. & White G. M. Observation and rehearsal as determinants of prosocial behavior. *Journal of Personality and Social Psychology,* 1967, **5,** 424–431.

Salomon, G. Cross-cultural distribution of television: A study of its effects on mental skills. Unpublished manuscript, Hebrew University of Jerusalem, 1974.

Shinar, D. Structure and content of television broadcasting in Israel. In G. A. Comstock & E. A. Rubinstein (eds.), *Television and social behavior. Vol. I: Media content and control.* Washington, D. C.: U.S. Government Printing Office, 1972, pp. 493–532.

Siegel, A. The influence of violence in the mass media upon children's role expectations. *Child Development,* 1958, **29,** 35–36.

Siegel, A. E. Film-mediated fantasy aggression and strength of aggressive drive. *Child Development,* 1956, **27,** 365–378.

Smythe, D. W. Reality as presented by television. *Public Opinion Quarterly,* 1954, **18,** 143–156.

Sprafkin, J. N., Liebert, R. M., & Poulos, R. W. Effects of a prosocial televised example on children's helping. *Journal of Experimental Child Psychology,* 1975, in press.

Stein. A. H. Mass media and young children's development. *71st Yearbook of the National Society for the Study of Education,* 1972, pp. 191–202.

Stein. A. H. & Friedrich, L. K, Television content and young chileren's behavior. In J. P. Murray, E. A. Rubinstein, & G. A. Comstock (eds.), *Television and social behavior. Vol. II: Television and social learning.* Washington, D.C.: U.S. Government Printing Office, 1972, pp. 202–317.

Stein. G. M. & Bryan, J. H. The effect of a televised model upon rule adoption behavior of children. *Child Development,* 1972, **43,** 268–273.

Sternglanz, S. H., & Serbin, L. A. Sex role stereotyping in children's television programs. *Developmental Psychology,* 1974, **10,** 710–715.

Steuer, F. B., Applefield, J. M. & Smith, R. Televised aggression and the interpersonal aggression of preschool children. *Journal of Experimental Child Psychology,* 1971, **11,** 442–447.

Time. The red tribe. January 12, 1968.

Tsai, M. K. Some effects of American television programs on children in Formosa. *Journal of Broadcasting,* 1969, **14,** 229–238.

Walters, R. H., Leat, M., & Mezei, L. Inhibition and disinhibition of responses through empathic learning. *Canadian Journal of Psychology,* 1963, **17,** 235–243.

Wolf, T. M., & Cheyne, J. A. Persistence of effects of live behavioral, televised behavioral, and live verbal models on resistance to deviation. *Child Development,* 1972, **43,** 1429–1436.

Yates, G. C. P. Influence of televised modeling and verbalisation on children's delay of gratification. *Journal of Experimental Child Psychology,* 1974, 18, 333–339.

Zajonc, R. Some effects on the "space" serials. *Public Opinion Quarterly,* 1954, **18,** 367–374.

Zimmerman, B. J., & Rosenthal, T. L. Observational learning of rule-governed behavior by children. *Psychological Bulletin,* 1974, **81,** 29–42.

PART TWO

Psychophysiologic and Behavior Disorders

CHAPTER 3

Childhood Asthma: The Role of Family Relationships, Personality, and Emotions*

KENNETH PURCELL

While the work of others will be cited, the intent of this paper is to present, in more or less integrated fashion, a summary of the principal investigations on psychological aspects of childhood asthma carried out by the author and his colleagues during the 1960s and early 1970s. The review outlines the development of our thinking as well as the empirical findings of various studies and their current relevance to clinical management and future research.

INITIAL OBSERVATION

One observation stimulated much of the research story that follows. This was the striking difference in symptom reaction noticed among severely asthmatic children who were admitted to the Children's Asthma Research Institute and Hospital (CARIH) in Denver from all parts of the United States. Some of these children (rapid remitters) became symptom free shortly after admission to CARIH and remained that way without regular medication for the 18–24 months of their residence. Others (termed steroid dependents) continued to have symptoms after admission to a degree that required constant maintenance doses of the powerful corticosteroid drugs for control. The central question that arose was, "What are the factors that account for this dramatic difference in symptom response to institutionalization?"

It seemed possible that one of the factors might be of a psychological nature. A number of other psychological investigations of asthma (e.g., Dubo, McLean, Ching, Wright, Kauffman, & Sheldon, 1961), often obtaining nega-

*Much of the author's work was supported by USPHS research grants MY3269, HD00884, MH08415, HD01060, and HD01529.

tive or inconclusive results, had grouped all asthmatics together, assuming that a fairly distinctive personality pattern or type of conflict was associated with the symptom. If some of these inconclusive results were a function of failure to discriminate important subgroupings within the asthmatic population, then a systematic attempt to classify asthmatics so as to determine the relative importance of allergic, emotional, and infectious stimuli should improve our understanding.

Most of the remainder of this paper describes the evolution of a research program aimed at discriminating between those children for whom psychological determinants play an important role in the maintenance of asthma and those for whom they do not, that is, the development of the asthma subgroup hypothesis. The determinants evaluated include parental attitude and personality, family relationships, child personality, and emotions. Studies will be discussed in roughly the chronological sequence in which they occured so that the thread of the investigation may be more easily followed. However, before reviewing the research trail that was followed, it may be helpful for the reader to learn something of the nature of asthma.

DESCRIPTION OF ASTHMA

Asthma is a symptom complex characterized by an increased responsiveness of the trachea, major bronchi, and peripheral bronchioles to various stimuli and manifested by extensive narrowing of the airways, which causes impairment of air exchange, primarily in expiration, and wheezing. A narrowing of the airway may be due to edema of the walls, increased mucous secretion, spasm of the bronchial muscles, or collapse of the posterior walls of the trachea and bronchi during certain types of forced expiration. The significance of these factors may vary from patient to patient and from attack to attack in the same patient. Similarly, the nature of the stimulation triggering these physiological processes may vary from patient to patient and attack to attack.

Hereditary Factors

Incidence of asthma in the families of asthmatic patients appears to be relatively high when compared with a similar group of nonasthmatic patients (Criep, 1962; Ratner & Silberman, 1953; Schwartz, 1952). However, it is also possible to find substantial numbers of asthmatics with essentially negative family histories. After surveying their own experience, Ratner and Silberman comment:

It seems to us, from the data of Schwartz, that what may be inherited is not the capacity to become sensitized (immunologically) but a respiratory tract which may react with the production of asthma or rhinitis due to a multiplicity of stimuli, one of which may be the antigen–antibody mechanism (1953, p. 374).

This hypothesis of organ vulnerability is similar to what is postulated for patients who may develop cardiovascular or gastrointestinal symptoms.

Incidence

The incidence of asthma in the population has been observed to be between 2.5 and 5% depending upon the method of estimate. A survey by the Public Health Service in 1957–1958 suggested that nearly 4,500,000 persons in this country were suffering from asthma at that time. About 60% of the population of asthmatics was below the age of 17. Asthma occurs in boys twice as often as among girls although the sex ratio evens out during the adult years. There are no well-documented explanations for this sex difference. Although asthma is relatively uncommon in infancy (Smyth, 1962), it has been diagnosed during the first few months of life and has been reported to start as late as the seventh decade.

Symptom Course

On the one hand, there is reason to be moderately optimistic about the future of a large percentage of asthmatic patients who first exhibit the symptom in childhood. Racheman and Edwards (1952) reviewed 449 patients who were first seen before 13 years of age and reevaluated 20 years later. Of the entire group, 71% had done extremely well with improvement generally beginning sometime during or soon after adolescence. On the other hand it is well to remember that asthma can be a life-threatening symptom. A report by Mustacchi, Lucia, and Jassy (1962) indicates that the fatality rate for this condition averages 1.5 deaths per 1000 asthmatic persons per year. Moreover, Gottlieb (1964) reports that, each year since 1949, from 4000 to nearly 7000 deaths in the United States were certified as primarily due to asthma. He notes that "asthma was noted in death certificates in 1960 about one-half as often as pulmonary tuberculosis, about one-third as often as malignant neoplasms of the lung, 8 times as often as menningococcal infections and 13 times as often as accidents to occupants of commercial aircraft" (p. 276).

Some indication of the socially disabling nature of the symptom is contained in the data of the United States National Health Survey indicating that in 1963 an average of about 64,000,000 days were lost to industry and schools because of asthma and hayfever. Asthma was estimated to be responsible for nearly one-fourth of the days reported lost from school because of chronic illness conditions in children (Schiffer & Hunt, 1963).

In general, unfavorable prognosis is associated with the older patient, disease of long duration, the presence of organic disease in the respiratory or circulatory organs, frequent and lengthy attacks, incomplete recovery between attacks, chronic cough, and failure to detect a "triggering stimulus."

Assessing the Symptom

Asthma is a highly unstable symptom that requires careful evaluation in order to obtain a reasonably accurate assessment of frequency and severity. The intermittent character of the symptom of asthma is dramatically shown in Figure 1, which compares a graph of expiratory peak flow rate obtained four times daily with less frequent measurements from the same patient. Some patients have long free periods between attacks. Others are chronically short of breath and begin wheezing very quickly in response to a whole array of stimuli, for example, exertion, dust, laughing hard, and so on.

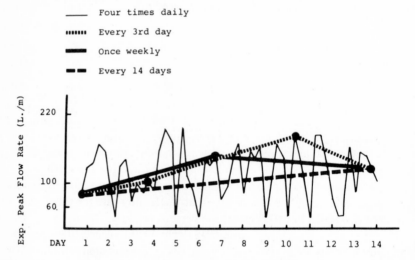

Figure 1.   Peak flow rates for 2 weeks in a 6-year-old boy. From K. Purcell et al. The effect of asthma in children of experimental separation from the family. *Psychosomatic Medicine,* 1969, **31,** No. 2, 150. Copyright 1969 by Harper & Row. Reprinted by permission.

An accurate estimate of frequency and severity of the symptom is important for several reasons, one of which is to assist in gauging the impact of the symptom on the psychological well being of the patient and his family. The inability to breathe is a frightening experience. Patients who have experienced severe episodes of asthma may be prone to panic reactions even during mild to moderate attacks. These panic states sometimes accentuate the respiratory difficulty. By way of contrast, teenage boys who wish to present a strong masculine image may underplay the severity of their symptoms. Such individuals frequently delay taking medication, or take reduced amounts in the effort to convince themselves that they are "normal." As might be expected, this type of defensive denial sometimes leads to serious and incapacitating asthmatic episodes.

Purcell, Brady, Chai, Muser, Molk, Gordon, and Means (1969), in a study assessing the effects of experimental separation from the family on asthmatic children, report a series of intercorrelations between the following four measures of asthma: (a) expiratory peak flow rate taken four times daily (the peak flow rate is perhaps the simplest of all the measures of lung function that the physician can obtain); (b) a physician's clinical examination scaling the severity of asthma at a given moment and done once daily; (c) daily history of a child's asthma as reported by his mother; (d) amount of medication administered to a child as reported by his mother.

The highest average correlation was between the history of severity of asthma and the amount of medication given (.60). This was not unexpected since each of these two measures described an entire 24-hour period as perceived by the same person, in this case a child's mother. The other measures were momentary: the clinical examination described the state of a child's symptom during a 1-minute period out of 24 hours and the average peak flow represented lung function during four 1-minute periods of the day. Of interest is the fact that the correlations between history of asthma and the amount of medication for individual subjects ranged from a low of .25 to a high of .85. The amount of medication taken by a child was, in a number of instances, determined by many factors, for example, fluctuating anxiety, symptom denial, and so on, other than simple symptom severity. Sometimes a parent adhered to a fixed quantity of medication regardless of symptom variability.

ASTHMA SUBGROUPS

Returning now to the problem that first caught our attention, how can we best understand the variability among asthmatics? In this section I describe three bases for subdivision that we have used in different studies. One involves the criterion of whether or not dramatic symptom change occurs following a child's departure from home and admission to a residential treatment center such as CARIH. The second, borrowed from other investigators, rests on a measure of organic vulnerability to allergic symptoms. Finally, we employed a psychological index, the Precipitant Interview, which seeks to measure the relative importance of different precipitants of asthma attacks as perceived by a child and/or his or her parents.

Symptom Response to Institutionalization

As noted earlier, we first compared subgroups that were defined on the basis of whether or not spontaneous remission of asthmatic symptoms occurred within a short time after admission to CARIH. Certain psychological differences between children, particularly between rapidly remitting and steroid-dependent groups, were found. For example, in response to a structured Precipitant Interview, rapidly remitting children reported significantly more often than did steroid-dependent children that emotions such as anger, anxiety, and depression triggered their asthma while at home (Purcell, 1963). Furthermore, the results of a questionnaire to assess parental child-rearing attitudes indicated that both mothers and fathers of rapidly remitting children showed authoritarian and punitive attitudes to a significantly greater degree than did the parents of steroid-dependent children (Purcell, Bernstein, & Bukantz, 1961).

We suggested the hypothesis that, among rapidly remitting children, in contrast to steroid-dependent children, the symptom of asthma is more often functionally linked with neurotic conflict and affective reactions. The asthmatic symptom of steroid-dependent children, on the other hand, was viewed as a response more regularly linked with influences of allergic and infectious factors. These differences between the two groups were regarded as relative rather than absolute.

Another study (Purcell & Metz, 1962) reported a substantial multiple correlation (.61) between two maternal attitude scales ("breaking the will" and "excluding outside influence") and age of onset of asthma in the rapidly remitting group, that is, the later the age of onset among children classified as rapid remitters, the higher the maternal score on these two variables. Age of onset ranged from birth to 5 years with a mean of 2.1 years. Within the steroid-dependent group, the corresponding multiple correlation was not significantly different from zero. These results were interpreted in two ways. First, and most generally, it was suggested that the finding of a statistically significant relationship between a psychologically defined variable (maternal attitudes) and an asthmatically defined variable (age of onset) in the rapidly remitting group but *not* in the steroid-dependent group was consistent with the hypothesis of psychological determinants having greater relevance for the former than for the latter group. Second, the homogeneity of the rapidly remitting group (with respect to any relationship between psychological variables and asthma) was questioned. We reasoned that autocratic and restrictive mothers (mothers of rapidly remitting children as contrasted to mothers of steroid-dependent children) pose no special problems for a dependent and confined infant for the first 12–18 months of life. However, with the development of a child's wishes for autonomy and independence, and with a broadening of his social world, autocratic maternal attitudes may make for serious conflicts between mother and child. For example, the period of toilet training often dramatizes the emergent clash of wills between mother and child. Similarly, the growing interest of the developing child in institutions and people outside the home creates particular difficulties for those mothers who feel it important to insulate their child from any outside influence that might lead the child to question his mother's authority. It is during this period of childhood stress that the rapidly remitting child may be highly motivated to learn to use the asthmatic response as a technique of coping with conflict.

If escape from a highly controlling, autocratic maternal relationship has something to do with symptom reduction in those rapid remitters with relatively late age of onset, for example, three to five years, then how may one account for improvement among remitters with a very early age of onset? It will be recalled that mothers of this latter group were considerably less autocratic and, therefore, symptom loss must be explained on some other basis. It may be that among these children removal from environmental allergens and/or climate variables are of particular importance. Results of an investigation (Purcell, Muser, Miklich, & Dietiker, 1969) bearing on this question of further refining the rapidly remitting classification are described later in this paper.

Allergic Potential Classification

Block, Jennings, Harvey, and Simpson (1964) challenged the assumption of homogeneity among asthmatic children by assessing a somatic variable. They subdivided asthmatic patients using an Allergic Potential Scale (APS) to evaluate a patient's predisposition to allergic reaction. The APS is based on such items as family history of allergy, skin test reactivity, eosinophile count, ease with which a particular symptom may be diagnosed as related to specific allergens, and total number of different organ systems involved in allergic reactions.

Using a thematic analysis of projective tests, these investigators concluded that the low APS children (less disposed to allergy but not significantly different from the high APS group on severity of asthma) were more pessimistic, conforming, and had lower frustration tolerance than the high APS children. Mothers and fathers independently described the low APS group more often as nervous, jealous, rebellious, and clinging, than the high APS group. The results of observations of mother–child interaction, quantified by an adjective Q-sort technique, indicated that mothers of low APS children were more

intrusive, angry, rejecting, and depriving. Scores on a parental attitude research questionnaire substantiated this evidence of undesirable maternal attitudes. Personality assessment of the mothers using the MMPI, TAT, and
Rorschach, suggested that mothers of the low APS children were more fearful,
anxious, and self-defeating with more evidence of psychopathology. Interviews
and observations of mother–father interaction indicated that the low APS
group of parents showed more ambivalent, destructive, and pathological relationships than the high APS group. To sum up, psychopathological factors
were observed significantly more often in low APS children and their mothers
than in high APS children and their mothers.

APS Scores and Symptom Response to Institutionalization

Finding that steroid-dependent and rapidly remitting children did not differ
in APS scores, we developed an hypothesis concerning the interaction between
these classificatory variables (Purcell, Muser, Miklich, & Dietiker, 1969). Our
thought was that children who are institutionalized generally experience a
major change in both their physically and psychologically defined environments. Symptom remission following institutionalization may be due to the
change in either class of stimuli or both. Those rapid remitters with high APS
scores represent children particularly predisposed to react with asthma to
allergic stimuli. Therefore, loss of symptoms in such cases may be principally
associated with alterations in surrounding allergic stimuli, whereas the low
APS rapid remitters may be responding more to the alteration in the psychological environment. One may expect to find, then, more evidence of parental
psychopathology, and perhaps of child psychopathology, in the low APS
remitters as compared to the high APS remitters.

Test data did indeed indicate the low APS remitters were significantly more
timid, anxious, depressed, and introverted than high APS remitters. Mothers
of low APS remitters appeared significantly more authoritarian, suppressive,
and intrusive than mothers of the high APS remitters. There were many more
significant differences associated with this breakdown of the subject population
than when either high and low APS groups or rapid remitter and steroid-
dependent groups were compared. Such differences were not found when low
APS steroid-dependents were compared with high APS steroid dependents.

These findings are consistent with the suggestion that the remission of
asthma symptoms following institutionalization may be a function of two
distinctive components: improvement associated with alteration of the total
physical environment to which the child is reactive and improvement associated with alteration of the psychological environment. Presumably the low
APS remitters, who displayed greater evidence of psychopathology and whose
mothers gave more indication of authoritarian-controlling attitudes toward
child rearing, may have responded with substantial changes in their emotional

status and in their learned behavior patterns to the massive changes in the psychological environment associated with institutionalization.

Infection is another biological pathway to asthma. In the study already cited (Purcell et al., 1969), two equally severe groups, one scoring high on *both* APS and URI (relevance of upper respiratory infection to asthma) and the other scoring low on APS and URI, were compared psychologically. Parents of children scoring low on both biological variables appeared more harsh, controlling, and restrictive in their child rearing attitudes than parents of the high–high group. The differences found when children were divided on the basis of APS alone were accentuated. In other words, when the contribution of a second biologically defined variable, upper respiratory infection, was added to the APS scores, the indication of controlling parental attitudes in the group with lower biological variable scores (low APS–low URI) was even clearer.

Experimental Separation of Asthmatic Children From Their Families

All of the above observations on symptom change associated with institutionalization involved removal of a child from his or her family home with accompanying changes in surrounding physical *and* psychological stimuli. The evidence implicating physical environmental factors in the perpetuation of asthma in certain children is quite clear. Therefore, if one is to isolate the effects of psychological variables it becomes of central importance to find a way of drastically altering the significant psychological environment with minimum modification of the physical environment.

Toward this end, we conducted an experiment (Purcell, Brady, Chai, Muser, Molk, Gordon, & Means, 1969) in which asthmatic children were studied medically and psychologically on a daily basis during periods in which they lived with their families and during an experimental 2-week period in which they had no contact with their families but were cared for in their own homes by a substitute parent. Every effort was made to maintain an essentially constant physical environment within the limits of normal variation. Children continued their normal daily activities, attended school, ate the same food as usual, etc.

The subjects were 25 chronically asthmatic, school-age children, living at home with their families in the Denver metropolitan community. Using the specially devised Precipitant Interview procedure these children were divided into two groups: (a) those for whom emotional factors appeared clinically to be highly relevant to asthma, and (b) those for whom emotional problems seemed irrelevant or less relevant. The former group (predicted positives) was expected to show an improvement in asthma during separation from their families; no improvement was anticipated in the latter group (predicted negatives). The experimental plan was divided into four 2-week periods labeled (a) qualification, (b) preseparation, (c) separation, and (d) reunion. Later, a fifth period, postreunion followup, was added for most subjects. During the qualification period, the family knew only that the investigators were engaging in a careful and intensive evaluation of asthma in children. Nothing was said about the possible separation. If the child met the requirements for frequency of asthma during the qualification period, the idea of separation was introduced as part of a thorough study of a difficult medical problem. Of 27 children satisfying all criteria and participating in the first 2 weeks of the experiment, 25 parents and children agreed to continue with the experiment after the separation concept was proposed.

Precipitant Interview

In previous work (Purcell, 1963) it was observed that children whose symptoms disappeared or diminished dramatically following admission to CARIH reported emotional precipitants to asthma attacks more often than children whose symptoms persisted to a degree requiring corticosteroid management. Since past experience suggested that reliable self-report was unlikely below age 8 or 9, and since a substantial number of children in the present study were younger than that, we decided to rely on parental observations. Thus, the interview for classifying subjects on the basis of predicted asthmatic response to separation was carried out with a child's parents *before* the beginning of the study.

Each parent was asked to list the things that he noticed brought on attacks of asthma in his child. It was emphasized that the interviewer was interested in what the parent himself noticed rather than what he might have heard from his physician, from other professionals, or from friends or relatives. Detailed information was collected on such items as the time interval between an event —be it damp weather or an argument—and the development of asthma. After a parent had spontaneously listed his observations, a list of additional asthma precipitants was read to him with the instruction that he indicate which, if any, applied to his child. The total list of items included the following: night asthma (unassociated in the parent's mind with any other precipitant); overexertion, weather (including change in season, dampness, heat, or cold), excitement (always with positive affect), emotional reactions (worry, upset, anger, sadness, or any other negative affects), laughing, crying, hard breathing, pollens (trees, grass, weeds), coughing, foods, colds, dust, other allergies, and "He just gets it."

After the listing was obtained, the parent was asked to rank the precipitants in their order of frequency in bringing on episodes of asthma. An estimate was obtained as to the absolute frequency with which a given precipitant was tied to the onset of asthma, for example, once a month, once a week, or less. Asking for illustrations of the operation of certain of the precipitants, for example, a description of the last time that your son was angry and you felt that this caused asthma, or that he ate a certain food which triggered asthma, was especially useful in assisting the parent to decide whether she was really reporting an occurrence from her own experience or merely parroting something heard from those around her. Vague reference to a possible link between emotions and the onset of asthma, for example, "Harriet is a nervous child and this probably affects her asthma," were not acceptable as precipitants unless supported by relatively clear examples of specific episodes.

Typically, seven to ten precipitants of asthma attacks were listed for each child. Children for whom emotions (anger, anxiety, excitement, depression) were ranked among the first three precipitants listed (by at least one and preferably both parents) in order of importance were predicted positives— those children whom we expected to improve during separation from the family. Those for whom emotions were not mentioned at all or were ranked among the least important precipitants were predicted negatives—those in whom improvement was *not* expected during separation. Other children, for whom emotions were ranked of middling importance, were not studied in this experiment.

Results

The basic question posed in this investigation was: "What is the effect on asthma of separating a child from his family while maintaining an essentially constant physical environment?" Therefore the main comparison was between the conditions of family-present and family-absent, that is, the qualification, the preseparation, and reunion periods combined versus the separation period. For the 13 predicted positive subjects, all measures of asthma—including expiratory peak flow rate, amount of medication required, daily history of asthma, and daily clinical examination—indicated that statistically significant improvement occurred during the period of family separation for the group as a whole. In contrast, only the daily history suggested improvement during separation for the 12 predicted negative subjects at a borderline level of statistical significance. Without corroboration from other measures, the daily history is a highly fallible, subjective indicator since a different adult observer (substitute parent) was involved during the separation as compared to the nonseparation periods.

The improvement in asthma during separation for the predicted positive group was fairly substantial, as judged by both the history of attacks and medication administered. Frequency of attacks was reduced, on the average, by well over half. This occurred while medication was being cut almost in half. There was also a highly significant 11% improvement in expiratory peak flow rate. Clinicians who are accustomed to thinking of a minimum 15–20% drop in forced expiratory volume as indicative of an attack of asthma may be misled by the 11% figure. One must remember that peak flows were collected at four standard times during the day whether or not a child was experiencing an attack of asthma. The great majority of these measurements were obtained in the absence of observable asthma. Under these conditions, an 11% increase is not only statistically, but also clinically, highly significant.

Comparisons were also carried out between the data of the qualification period and the separation period. As will be recalled, the qualification period represented the initial 2-week baseline period. The pattern of findings was virtually identical to that found when all three periods of family presence were combined. As a matter of secondary interest, a similar analysis was carried out comparing the qualification with the preseparation period. Psychoanalytic theorists (French & Alexander, 1941) have suggested that threat of separation may be an important stimulus to the provocation of asthmatic symptoms. The qualification period was one in which neither family or child was aware of any possible separation while the preseparation period was characterized by knowledge of the impending separation by all parties. None of the differences between these periods achieved statistical significance for either the predicted positive or predicted negative group. In other words, threat of separation, as defined in this experiment, did not increase asthmatic symptoms.

Figures 2–5, showing the period by period changes in asthma, probably best illustrate the impact of the separation. The mean scores for each experimental period for each asthmatic index are presented in Figures 2–5 for the predicted positive group. It is clear that not only was separation associated with a fairly sharp reduction of symptoms but that within 2 weeks after the family returned home these children showed an increase in asthma symptoms approaching the preseparation levels. During separation, the expiratory peak flow rate improved and there was less clinical evidence of asthma despite the fact that the children received substantially *less* antiasthmatic medication during separation. These means are quite stable as the score for each 2-week period represents many observations. For example, each 2-week score for peak flow is the mean of 728 observations, 13 children × 56 observations per child (4 per day for 14 days). Again, corresponding figures for the predicted negative group failed to reveal any pattern of change in asthma associated with separation.

Family and Personality Data

Simultaneous with the measurements of asthma, several kinds of psychological information were gathered (Purcell, 1973). These included structured interviews and certain standard tests. Interviews with both children and parents were conducted at fixed points in the experimental sequence and tape recorded.

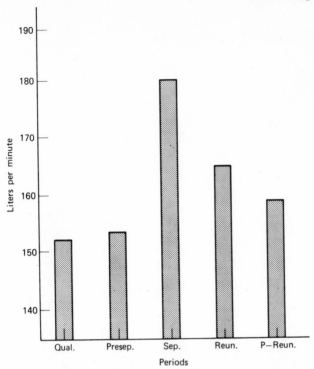

Figure 2.   Mean daily expiratory peak flow rate for predicted positive group ($N = 13$) during each period of study. From K. Purcell et al. The effect of asthma in children of experimental separation from the family. *Psychosomatic Medicine,* 1969, **31,** No. 2, 153. Copyright 1969 by Harper & Row. Reprinted by permission.

However, the interviews with children did not contain enough material for analysis. The two most important parental interviews (both parents together) focused on anticipated and actual reactions to the separation. The first interview (Interview A) analyzed was conducted 2 weeks after the study began and was the one in which the investigators first broached the idea of experimental separation to the parents. The second interview (Interview B) took place 2 days after the beginning of the separation.

Interview A was coded for ten variables: pleasure that parents expect from separation, pain and discomfort that parents expect during separation, parents' concern over their role in the child's asthma, parents' expression of how they would miss their child, parents' perception of child's demands for attention, degree of parental overprotectiveness, parents' readiness to accept responsibility for preparing the child for separation, parents' impression of child's asthma during previous separations, parents' report about the ease with which previ-

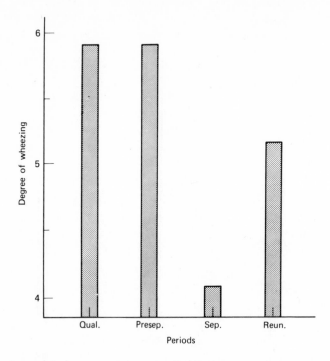

Figure 3. Mean daily scores for clinical evidence of wheezing for predicted positive group ($N=13$) during each period of study. *Children did not make daily visits to institute for examination in postreunion period. From K. Purcell et al. The effect of asthma in children of experimental separation from the family. *Psychosomatic Medicine,* 1969, **31**, No. 2, 153. Copyright 1969 by Harper & Row. Reprinted by permission.

ous separations were accomplished, and parents' report of child's adjustment to previous separations.

Interview B was coded for a somewhat different set of variables: parents' pleasurable experiences during separation, parents' pain or discomfort during separation, parents' expression of how much they missed their child, parents' perception of child's demand for attention at the time of separation, amount of parental attention to and "fussing over" the child at the time of leave taking, degree of parental overprotectiveness at the time of separation, parents' report about the ease of separation for the child, parental reaction at the time of separation, parental anxiety over the child's welfare, and parental impression of the degree to which the child appeared disturbed during the separation (the latter was based on the parents' interpretation of conversations with the substitute parent or sometimes neighbors).

Interview A results indicated that mothers of predicted positive children were rated as differing from mothers of predicted negative children on six of ten scales. For example, they anticipated missing their child more, felt that previous leave takings were difficult, felt that their child tended to be upset during past separations, and showed a relative lack of willingness to assume responsibility for preparing the child for the forthcoming separation. The same pattern of data was apparent for fathers, although to a somewhat lesser degree. Similar differences were evident after the first 2 days of separation. Parents of predicted positive children, as compared to parents of predicted negative children, appeared to be suffering more, to feel their child needed them more, to have missed their child more, and to have had a somewhat more difficult time parting from their child. The differences after separation were more numerous and substantial than the differences before separation suggesting that, in this instance, the reality was experienced more keenly than the anticipation.

Test data comparing predicted positive and predicted negative groups yielded relatively few significant differences, but these were consistent with data already reported. In 13 Parental Attitude Research Instrument (PARI) scale comparisons (Zuckerman, 1959) the groups were significantly different from one another on two, "intrusiveness" and "rejection of the homemaking role." The intrusiveness scale was made up of items such as "a mother has a right to know everything going on in her child's life because her child is part of her," and the rejection of homemaking role contained items such as "most mothers are content to be with children all the time." Mothers of predicted positives scored higher on the intrusiveness and lower on rejection of homemaking than mothers of predicted negatives.

On the MMPI scales, fathers of predicted positives scored higher on the Psychopathic Deviate and Psychoasthenia scales than did fathers of predicated negatives. There were no significant differences between mothers on any of the clinical scales. Nor was there any significant difference between predicted positive and predicted negative groups in scores on a behavior problem checklist. Both mothers and fathers described these two groups as having about the same number of behavioral problems, past and present.

None of the 16 IPAT (Porter & Cattell, 1960) test score differences was large enough to attain significance. There was some tendency for predicted positive children to score higher than predicted negative children on the Children's Manifest Anxiety Scale (Castaneda, McCandless, & Palermo, 1956).

Clearly, the parents of the predicted positive group, particularly mothers, reported being more upset and concerned about their children than did parents of the predicted negative group. Before discussing the implications of this finding, it seems worth examining some possible artifactual sources of the group differences. For example, if the groups were different in severity of

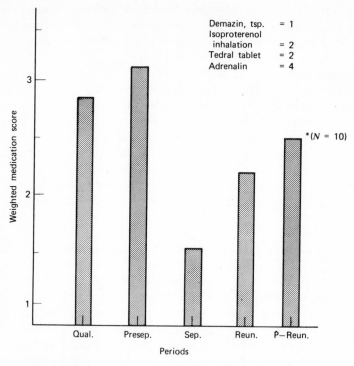

Figure 4.   Mean daily medication scores for predicted positive group ($N=13$) during each period of study. *Data collection during postreunion period was not begun until after first few subjects were completed. From K. Purcell et al. The effect of asthma in children of experimental separation from the family. *Psychosomatic Medicine,* 1969, **31,** No. 2, 153. Copyright 1969 by Harper & Row. Reprinted by permission.

asthma, there might be an objective basis for greater concern on the part of one set of parents. The children, however, did not differ on this variable. Second, there exists the possibility that parents of predicted positives simply tended to talk more about psychological difficulties than parents of predicted negatives. After all, the parents of predicted positives were also the ones who reported more evidence of emotional precipitants of asthma for their children. If, however, this were the case, one would expect evidence of this tendency to show up in other data, for example, the number of behavior problems checked by parents on the behavior problem checklist. There were no significant differences between the two groups in the number of behavior problems noted.

Assuming that the interview differences are genuine, that is, that, in response to separation, there was a greater degree of anxious concern among parents of predicted positives, how might this be interpreted? The results are consistent with the possibility that asthma may be maintained in at least some children by a learning process involving parental reinforcement of the symptom. If we postulate that asthma is, in part, maintained by family reinforcements, removal of the child from that family should disrupt these reinforcement contingencies. Of course, the results simply suggest a parental, and particularly maternal, focus of attention on the child with asthma that is substantially greater in the group that improved during separation than in the other group. While these results fit in very well with the PARI findings that mothers of predicted positives intrude more in their children's lives and are more deeply involved in the homemaking role, they do not clearly demonstrate that asthma is maintained by the reinforcer of parental attention at the time asthma occurs.

The psychological differences between parental groups may influence the course of asthma via a respondent process as well as an operant (reinforcement) one. Not uncommonly, aversive reinforcement produces an emotional respondent, which in turn elicits asthma. For example, in the course of daily reporting on the precipitants of asthma attacks in her child, Mrs. R. became aware that asthma was sometimes contingent on certain behavioral events. She made this observation at the end of the study: "You know how Mike used to have asthma at almost every meal when I tried to get him to eat. I'd scold him and he would get angry and choke up and then start to cough and then, bingo, he would have asthma. Well, I decided if Mike didn't finish his food we would just leave him at the table to clean up the dishes and not say anything. Since we started that he hasn't coughed once at mealtime—and no asthma at those times." By not saying anything and leaving Mike alone at the table, Mrs. R. disrupted the usual chain of events by removing the cues for punishment during mealtime. Consequently Mike's anger, and the respiratory behaviors often associated with his anger, that is, choking and coughing, did not occur. As pointed out by Purcell (1963) and Purcell and Weiss (1970), such respiratory activity may lead to airway narrowing by reflex mechanisms.

A different type of respondent behavior may be seen in the following episode: Two subjects were brothers, and, on the basis of initial interviews, one child, Harry, was selected as a predicted positive and the other boy, Joey, as a predicted negative. The studies were carried out sequentially and Harry's asthma did improve during separation while Joey's did not. The substitute mother, Miss K., who stayed with Harry was a trained nurse and careful observer. She reported, and we confirmed in our own interviews, that the boy's mother was a compulsively meticulous housekeeper who made a ritual of keeping everything around her spotless, furniture, carpets, children, and so on. Joe was described as a terror who was afraid of nothing. His mother's critical remarks were said to "roll off his skin like water off a duck's back." Harry, on the other hand, was said to be much more sensitive and attached to his mother. During the 2 weeks of separation Harry was entirely free of asthma except for a single 1-minute period of very mild wheezing. One evening Miss K. had some guests visiting her and noticed Harry standing hesitantly at the foot of the stairway. To quote Miss K., "I went up to him and he was shivering and hyperventilating very hard and looked scared to death. There was just the start of a wheeze I could hear. He told me he had had an accident, wet his pants—and some had got on the carpet. I told him we could fix that easily and calmed him and I was amazed. In less than 60 seconds his breathing was back to normal, no more wheezing and he didn't need a nebulizer." One may conceptualize this episode as a conditioned anxiety reaction of which asthma was a correlate. Again, the respiratory tract stimulation produced by hyperventilation may have triggered reflex airway constriction.

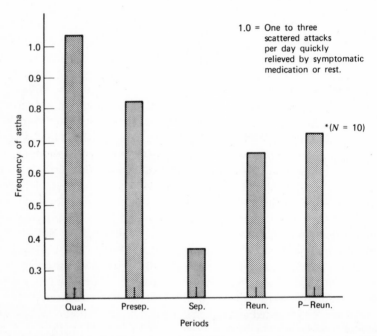

Figure 5. Mean daily frequency of asthma for predicted positive group ($N=13$) during each period of study. *Data collection in the postreunion period was not begun until after the first few subjects were completed. From K. Purcell et al. The effect of asthma in children of experimental separation from the family. *Psychosomatic Medicine,* 1969, **31**, No. 2, 153. Copyright 1969 by Harper & Row. Reprinted by permission.

In summary, the suggestion conveyed by these two examples is that parental attitudes and/or techniques of managing behavior may influence asthma by influencing the frequency of occurrence of emotional events that precipitate asthma.

MECHANISMS FOR THE OPERATION OF PSYCHOLOGICAL VARIABLES

Until the experimental separation study we had largely been concentrating on relating personality and attitudinal measures to asthmatic subgroup differences with the implicit assumption that somehow these personality and attitudinal variables mediated the differences in asthmatic response to instutionalization. Exploration of these variables continued in the separation study but, in addition, the role of emotional states began to come to the forefront in our thinking. This resulted in part from the fact that interview assessment of the importance of emotional states as triggers of asthma clearly predicted improvement during experimental separation from the family. Moreover, because of the close, continuous observation of children during that study, we learned of a number of incidents (such as the two just cited) that compellingly suggested the importance of emotions. Therefore, our next major effort was to attempt to gain more direct information about the part played by emotional states. Before describing this work it might again be useful to digress in order to outline the pathways through which emotional states might influence asthma as well as to review briefly the evidence implicating other psychological variables such as personality types or specific forms of conflict.

There are a variety of mediating mechanisms through which emotional states may influence asthma. First, autonomic activity associated with emotional arousal can initiate the airway obstruction characteristic of an asthmatic attack by stimulating mucous secretion, vascular engorgement, or bronchial constriction. For example, it is known that vagal stimulation produces rapid bronchospasm and secretion. Second, emotional states are often associated with certain respiratory behaviors, for example, crying, laughing, coughing, hyperventilation, which can lead to airway narrowing by reflex mechanisms. In these cases, a vagal reflex arch may be activated by the stimulation of subepithelial cough receptors (Simonsson, Jacobs, & Nadel, 1967). The autonomic discharge and the respiratory mechanisms mediating the effects of emotions are by no means mutually exclusive. Hyperventilation, for example, may occur in association with certain emotional states and patterns of autonomic arousal. Or autonomic activity may initiate mucous secretion, provoking a cough followed by reflex bronchoconstriction. Third, emotions have been shown to influence significantly endogenous adrenal steroid output (Hamburg, 1962; Handlon, Wadeson, Fishman, Sacher, Hamburg, & Mason, 1962), which may, in turn, alter the course of asthma. Reinberg (1963), for example, has reported data suggesting some correspondence between the occurrence of nocturnal asthma attacks and the nightly periodic decrease in adrenocortical activity. Fourth, the physiological responses of mucous secretion, bronchospasm, or vascular engorgement may, through learning, be increased in intensity and duration to the point of inducing significant airway obstruction. Finally, it is possible, but not yet demonstrated, that central nervous system processes may influence the immunologic phenomena (antigen–antibody reactions) producing tissue change associated with narrowing of the airways.

There is one other particularly interesting possibility for an indirect mode of action of emotions. It happens that upper respiratory infections are an important and common trigger of asthmatic attacks. The majority of respiratory infections have their origin in viral invasion of the organism with bacteria also gaining entrance through tissues already damaged by viral penetration (Proctor, 1964). In order for a virus to penetrate a cell there must be contact between the virus and cell wall for an appreciable period of time. Frequently viruses and bacteria that are contained in inspired air are trapped in nasal mucous, swept away by ciliary action, and disposed of in the stomach without any cell penetration. However, if the cilia-propelled mucous blanket is not functioning normally then the virus may become lodged on a mucosal surface long enough for penetration and infection to occur. A number of different internal and external influences may affect mucosal function, both secretion and ciliary action. Among these influences are controls mediated through the neuroendocrine and autonomic nervous systems. It appears possible that various forms of emotional expression may act through these systems to affect both the nasal mucous membrane and the mucous membranes of the tracheobronchial tree in ways which would increase the likelihood of viral cell penetration and subsequent upper respiratory infection.

Is There a Personality Constellation or Nuclear Conflict Specific to Asthmatics?

Out of a large body of literature, mainly descriptive and nonexperimental case studies, had come suggestions regarding a common personality profile descriptive of asthmatic patients or a specific type of nuclear conflict, for example, unresolved dependency on the mother, as especially applicable to asthmatics. Many authors implied that these characteristics bear a causal relationship to the development of the asthmatic symptom; others noted that they appeared secondary, resulting from the symptom and its effects on the patient and his family. Asthmatics, particularly children, were described as anxious, dependent, conforming, insecure, lacking in self-confidence, and hypersensitive. Our own view was that a careful examination of the literature did not suggest that any specific personality constellation, nuclear conflict, or form of inter-personal relationship is uniformly and etiologically associated with asthma. This assertion, which does not deny the observation that asthmatics and their families often manifest more behavioral disturbance than normal subjects, was based on the following lines of evidence.

Neuhaus (1958) found that both asthmatic and cardiac patients (children) were significantly more maladjusted (anxious, insecure, and dependent) than a normal control group but did not differ from each other. He concluded that chronic illness may be the variable most relevant to the production of behavioral maladjustment in asthmatics rather than some process associated specifically with asthma. Furthermore, our own work (Purcell, Turnbull, & Bernstein, 1962) failed to disclose any differences between asthma subgroups in personality profile or degree of neuroticism. What differences there were emerged from an examination of specific relationships between psychological variables and asthma, for example, perceived precipitants of asthma, as opposed to global personality measurement using standard diagnostic tests.

A suggestion that unresolved dependency conflicts are central in the development of asthma is contained in the influential writings of French and Alexander (1941), who further hypothesize that asthma may often be viewed as a suppressed cry, with the stated implication that asthmatic children cry less than nonasthmatics, particularly around critical periods of separation conflict. To our knowledge, there was no systematic survey of crying behavior to support this assertion. Nevertheless, clinicians had sometimes noted a tendency for crying to be distorted in a silent, awkward way in certain of their patients. Purcell (1963) had suggested an alternative interpretation of this observation, noting that a number of patients report that crying, like laughing and coughing, can trigger attacks of asthma and further, that these patients sometimes deliberately seek to avoid crying or laughing hard so as not to provoke asthma. Thus, the occasionally observed inability to cry or the silent, suppressed manner of crying may simply reflect a learned attempt to avoid initiating the uncomfortable experience of an asthmatic attack.

At this stage, then, our review of research studies and of our own experience led to the overriding impression that the kinds of behavioral antecedents most immediately relevant to asthma were emotional states rather than attitudes or patterns of interpersonal relationship. These latter variables may be thought of as distal antecedents since it is certainly quite plausible that they affect the type, frequency, intensity and duration of emotional states.

Emotions and Asthma

Having selected emotional states as a key psychological variable, the question arose as to when and where these were to be studied. Too often we seemed ready to assume a clear and direct link between an emotional problem and a clinical syndrome. That is, one might see an emotionally disturbed asthmatic child or family and assume that the emotional disturbance was necessarily relevant to asthma. The point, which has been made elsewhere, is that a personality description may be perfectly accurate, yet etiologically and functionally unrelated to the specific disorder presented by the child. These considerations led us away from studies of the general emotional constellation in a child and his or her family to a focus on the antecedents and concomitants of the particular response in which we were interested, the asthmatic attack. The logic underlying this approach states that if emotions are important in producing asthma, it should be possible to demonstrate a specific role for such variables in the precipitation of individual attacks.

Moreover, we felt that if we were to learn something of the importance of any functional relationship between emotional states and asthma in life situations, for example, its frequency of occurrence, we must study it naturalistically in the context of life situations. It is, for example, quite conceivable that asthma might be experimentally induced by affective stimuli that might nevertheless play an exceedingly minor role in the triggering of asthma during the normal life of that child. Freeman, Feingold, Schlesinger, and Gorman (1964) had noted that "most work in this area has suffered from major methodological problems in obtaining pertinent and reliable information about life circumstances at the time of onset of symptoms" (p. 567). Our plan sought to overcome this defect by obtaining a complete, accurate, and simultaneous record of spontaneously occuring asthma and vocal behavior in the daily life of a child. These needs dictated a choice of a miniature radio transmitter worn by the child as the medium for collecting data. The entire transmitter output (both respiratory sounds and all vocal behavior) would be tape recorded at a remotely located receiving station. Such data should permit a more comprehensive and precise description of the psychological events preceding and accompanying spontaneous attacks of asthma than had previously been available.

Method Issues

Before proceeding with the main study, it was necessary to develop data bearing on some methodological questions. Our initial aims were (a) to assess the effects of the observational technique (constant monitoring by a radio transmitter) upon the behavior obtained. Would the subjects adapt to the procedure and behave naturally?; (b) to attempt an estimate of the kind and quantity of interpersonal communication that is missed by a technique relying exclusively upon auditory observation.

We found (Purcell & Brady, 1966) that within a short time (usually no more than 2–4 days) children appeared to behave quite naturally as judged by all of the following indices: (a) direct measures of attention to the transmitting system as scored from tape recorded verbal behavior, (b) subjective reports of the children, (c) observations by the cottage house parents. Furthermore, assessment of interpersonal behavior based on sound recording alone appeared to yield about as much usable information as sound recording plus visual data such as descriptions of gesture, expression, and so on obtained in the form of a specimen record by an observer present at the time of the original interaction.

Initially, our system of analysis was designed to describe interpersonal behavior patterns. Papers by Purcell and Brady (1965; 1966) present in detail the scoring system, the data relevant to methodological issues, and some preliminary information on the utility and validity of the data gathered. Later, using the same transmitter gathered data, we conducted interscorer reliability studies for various categories of emotion (anger, depression, excitement, and anxiety) and respiratory behavior (laughing, yelling, crying, coughing, and hyperventilation). Interjudge agreement coefficients for all of these averaged over .90 with none being lower than .83.

Our original plan had been to use a two-channel miniature radio transmitter with one channel recording the sounds of respiration and the other channel recording the vocal behavior of the child and others in the immediate vicinity. We wished to compare the incidence and intensity of emotional states and certain vocal behaviors prior to asthma with their occurrence during equivalent nonasthma control periods. Operationally, this meant scoring a 30-minute period before the onset of wheezing and selecting a comparable 30-minute period (same time of day, same setting) that was not followed by asthma.

Unfortunately, because of the number of technical problems surrounding the recording of respiration, we had to change our plan for gathering these data. In place of the telemetric recording of the respiration, measures were taken of expiratory peak flow function every 20 minutes. Expiratory peak flow rates, as noted earlier, are easily obtained by having the child blow into a small, portable apparatus weighing about one pound. A research assistant regularly recorded these measurements for a subject approximately every 20 minutes from the time the child returned from school until bedtime. Such an arrangement was possible because of the fact that the study took place in a residential treatment and research center where the children spent most of their time. A total of 18 boys, ranging in age from 10 years, 6 months to 14 years, 10 months, were studied for an average duration of 3–4 weeks each (Miklich, Chai, Purcell, Weiss, & Brady, 1974).

We did succeed in monitoring voice interactions reasonably successfully over a 15-acre area and for about 5 hours daily, the period between the end of school and bedtime. However, because of the varying availability of children as well as technical problems associated with the radiotelemetry system (Miklich, Purcell, & Weiss, in press), considerably fewer than 5 hours daily of tape were scorable. For the 20 minutes preceding every peak flow measurement we computed a composite score reflecting the frequency, intensity, and duration of each emotion and vocal behavior, for example, laughing, that occurred in that 20-minute period. These scores for each emotion and vocal behavior were then correlated with the peak flow measurements taken at the end of the 20-minute period.

Results

Certain emotions (depression, anxiety) and vocal behaviors (crying, hyperventilation) occurred too infrequently to be meaningfully analyzed. Thus, we were left with anger, excitement, yelling, and laughing as variables that were coded with sufficient frequency to be related to changes in lung function. Table 1 shows the correlations with peak flow measurements.

Table 1.   Correlations of Emotions and Vocal Behaviors with Peak Flow Rates

Subject	N^a	Vocal Behaviors		Emotions	
		Laughing	Yelling	Anger	Exitement
1	44	−.44 [b]	−.04	.20	.08
2	188	−.16 [c]	−.05	−.10	−.07
3	120	−.14	.11	−.02	.03
4	128	−.27 [b]	−.12	.01	−.04
5	71	−.01	−.12	.13	No data
6	132	−.05	.01	−.10	−.16 [c]
7	45	−.02	.17	.06	.11
8	39	−.40 [b]	−.47 [b]	−.29 [c]	−.59 [b]
9	162	.09	.08	.03	.15
10	145	−.27 [b]	.04	.09	−.09
11	48	.19	−.21	−.05	−.10
12	103	−.12	−.01	.05	−.02
13	37	−.42 [b]	−.34 [c]	−.19	.18
14	64	−.13	.06	.02	.01
15	22	−.27	.01	−.58 [b]	.35
16	132	−.22 [2]	−.27 [b]	−.07	−.23 [b]
17	100	−.23 [c]	−.12	−.27 [b]	.01
18	63	.11	.01	−.10	.19

[a] N^a refers to number of available and scorable 20 minute tape segments for a subject.
[b] Significantly different from zero at < .01 level.
[c] Significantly different from zero at < .05 level.

Seven of the boys showed a pattern of more intense laughter followed by lower peak flows. Three also showed peak flow drops following yelling. It appears, therefore, that increases in the vocal behaviors of yelling and laughing can trigger decreases in flow rates and presumably, therefore, precipitate asthma. Anger was followed by lower peak flows among three boys as was excitement. A total of five boys developed lower peak flows following emotional arousal, one boy showing the relationship with both anger and excitement. While the correlations involving emotions are not frequent, in at least two cases they are surprisingly large and, in fact, are larger than any of the laughing or yelling correlations.

The question arises as to whether the relationships between emotions and lung function were mediated by laughing and yelling behavior. It appears not. If laughing or yelling were the mediating variables we would expect the correlations with these vocal behaviors to be larger than the same boys' correlations with emotions. However, the correlations between peak flow and emotions for those boys were as large and often larger than the correlations involving vocal behaviors. Moreover, when the effects of vocal behaviors were partialled out, using a partial correlation technique, the size of the correlation between peak flow and emotions did not change.

A few other observations about these data, which are not yet completely analyzed, may be appropriate. First, for a given subject, emotional triggering of lowered peak flow appeared to occur only when emotional arousal was relatively intense. However, the degree of emotional arousal was sometimes less than that which another boy might exhibit without triggering a drop in flow rate. Thus it is not the intensity of emotional arousal alone that is capable of producing asthma in any boy. Rather, there is likely a learned association between emotion and alteration in lung function among those susceptible to emotional triggering. Further, the size in the drop of flow rate (over 15%) which was associated with intense emotion in certain children was of sufficient magnitude to be indicative of clinical asthma.

Second, we were interested in examing whether those children for whom emotion–lung function relations were found might also be children characterized by psychopathological adjustment. Clinical psychologists independently rated the psychological adjustment of each of the 18 subjects in this study. Each of the five boys for whom we found an emotion–peak flow correlation was considered to be of average or better than average adjustment. On the other hand, none of the four boys who were judged as having the worst adjustment showed any signs of emotionally triggered peak flow drops. These four maladjusted boys were studied much longer than the other subjects. They showed many emotions, but these emotions were not followed by reduced peak flows. Thus, it appears that psychological maladjustment, in and of itself, has little to do with whether or not emotional states tend to influence the occurrence of asthma.

Finally, a growing body of evidence referred to elsewhere in this paper suggests that a carefully structured precipitant interview may provide the best information as to whether psychological factors are of significance in triggering asthma for a particular child. Unfortunately, there were certain difficulties in collecting these data at CARIH that made for imperfect relationships between the precipitant interview data and the emotion–peak flow correlations. The main problem was that only one of the children reported any emotional precipitants of asthma while at CARIH whereas 13 of them reported such precipitants when they were living at home. Thus, the study data were gathered in a residential setting which was very different from the home setting and in which emotional precipitant reports were rare as compared to home. This led to 9 of 13 false positives, that is, emotional precipitants reported in the interview but not found in the study. Of five children not reporting emotional precipitants, one was a false negative, that is, showed a significant emotion–peak flow correlation. These numbers are too small to weight heavily but it does appear likely that in the different environment of a residential treatment center certain emotional reactions might not have occurred as frequently or as intensely as at home. Some support for this suggestion is found in the fact that we did not observe sufficient amounts of anxiety to justify analysis of this variable although 7 of the 18 children reported anxiety as capable of precipitating asthma at home. It may well be that the extent of emotional triggering of asthma in this study is a conservative estimate of that which occurs when the child is in his home environment.

In summary, therefore, it appears that emotions of anger and excitement and the vocal behaviors of yelling and laughing were all capable of independently triggering peak flow rate decreases and presumably triggering asthma. The emotional triggering did not appear to be especially frequent and occurred in only some subjects. The boys for whom it did occur were not characterized by especially intense or frequent emotional outbursts in comparison with other boys nor did they exhibit any special degree of psychological maladjustment.

IMPLICATIONS OF THE SUBGROUP HYPOTHESIS

Cues for Clinical Management

In light of the results described above, how may the clinician approach the evaluation of the relevancy of psychological factors for the particular asthmatic patient with whom he must deal? The tools and cues found most useful clinically are those that have successfully, albeit imperfectly, discriminated among asthmatic subgroups. There are four classes of information involved: (a) the patient's, or in the case of a child below the age of eight or nine, his parents', perception of events related to the onset of asthma attacks; (b) the nature of the symptom response to separation from significant figures; (c) biological characteristics of the patient; (d) presence of certain attitudes and/or degree of psychopathology in the parent and child. These are briefly discussed in sequence.

Information on perceived precipitants of attacks may be obtained from the Precipitant Interview, which fairly successfully distinguished rapid remitters from steroid-dependent children and predicted improvers and nonimprovers in the experimental separation study. A practical rule of thumb is to consider psychological variables relevant to the maintenance of asthma when emotions such as anger, anxiety, excitement, or depression are ranked among the first three precipitants of asthma in order of importance by either the patient or his parents and when specific episodes supporting this ranking can be given by the informant. Two recent reports by different investigators provide further validating evidence for the precipitant interview. Miklich, Rewey, Weiss, and Kolton (1973) found the interview useful in evaluating psychophysiological responses to stress. Variables studied were heart rate, finger pulse amplitude, respiration durations and rates, and peak expiratory flow rates. Stress was induced by arbitrarily criticizing asthmatic boys for their performance on mental arithmetic problems. Marked effects were evident for all variables except the peak expiratory flow rate. Asthmatics reporting emotional precipitants of asthma showed abnormal respiration patterns and reduced vasoconstriction to the stress as compared to asthmatics not reporting emotional precipitants. Alexander (1973) also employed the precipitant interview in a study of systematic relaxation and its effect on respiration in asthmatic children. He found that relaxation training produced greater improvement in expiratory flow rates among subjects reporting emotional precipitants of asthma than among those who did not.

Changes in symptoms associated with separation from parents or siblings may occur in several different situations. For example, a very prompt response to hospitalization without the use of any potent medication is a frequent report. Parents have reported in the case of some children that there is a consistent improvement as the child reaches the vicinity of the hospital even before getting to the emergency room. It is useful to inquire closely about the course of asthma during those periods when a child has been separated from one or both of his parents in the normal course of events. For example, husbands may go off on business trips or parents may take vacations for a few days or more at a time leaving their child with a babysitter. The clinician must always keep in mind that separation from significant persons is frequently accompanied by a change in the physical environment, which itself may be associated with alterations in asthmatic symptoms. Often it is not possible to do much more than make an educated guess as to which factors are primarily responsible for a symptom change. When fairly unambiguous data are available on this point, for example, a child repeatedly improving during separation from his family with any accompanying changes in the physical environment appearing insignificant, it deserves to be heavily weighted in evaluating the role of psychological variables.

Much of the historical information on biological characteristics can be obtained directly by the psychologically oriented clinician. However, some of it must be sought from the physician involved in the case. The strength of constitutional disposition toward allergy varies directly with the degree of positive finding in APS items such as family history of allergy, total number of allergies in the patient, ease of diagnosability of specific allergens, and skin test reactivity. Unfortunately, quantitative data describing cut off scores for judging the significance of APS scores are not available.

Indications of highly controlling, autocratic maternal attitudes may point to the operation of psychological variables. However, it is likely that, when these attitudes are clearly relevant to the maintenance of asthma, one should also find more direct evidence of emotions triggering attacks or of asthma remitting upon separation from such a mother.

Sheer degree of psychopathology in the child is, in the writer's judgment, the least valuable cue. For one thing, the evidence on this point is ambiguous. While one study (Block et al., 1964) reported differences between asthmatic subgroups in overall degree of psychopathology, another (Purcell & Turnbull, 1962) did not. Even more important are data (Neuhaus, 1958) suggesting that behavioral maladjustment among asthmatics is no different than maladjustment found among children suffering from cardiac defects, with both groups differing from the normal. Therefore, even when one finds important indications of emotional disturbance in the child, these may be more the consequences of a chronic illness condition than the antecedents of asthma.

A cautionary note in evaluating all these indices is the fact that asthma is almost always a multiply triggered symptom. In the individual case, asthma precipitated by physically defined stimuli almost invariably coexists with asthma precipitated by psychologically defined stimuli. Therefore, a seemingly high score on biological characteristics does not preclude the possibility that emotional stimuli are important, with the reverse being true as well.

At the least, the results obtained from subgroup studies offer some assistance in making a more informed judgment about whether or not to include some form of psychotherapeutic intervention as part of the treatment program for asthma. The information most useful in guiding clinical decisions at this time is probably that dealing with emotional precipitants of asthma attacks and the effects of separation from family members on asthma.

Research Implications

Asthma is conceptualized as a symptom arising from an overreactivity of the respiratory apparatus (probably on an hereditary basis) to a multiplicity of stimuli, for example, infections, psychological, immunologic. As interpreted by the present author the subgroup hypothesis assumes, first, that in the typical cases attacks of asthma are usually triggered by a variety of stimuli. Second, there is no logical or empirical requirement that, because one class of stimuli frequently triggers attacks for a given individual, we must then necessarily assume the other classes of stimuli are less important. A severe asthmatic may have attacks equally frequently instigated by all classes of stimuli. Only when one is comparing individuals or groups *equated* for symptom severity does it appear sensible that, if emotional stimuli are high in relevance to asthma for one group and low for another, then the reverse should be true among one or more of the remaining stimulus classes.

Any investigation that fails to discriminate among asthmatics runs the risk of obscuring relationships that may exist only for a portion of the population. For example, using a population of 71 ambulant children with chronic asthma, Dubo et al. (1961) tested the hypothesis of a positive relationship between disturbances in family dynamics and severity of asthma in a child. They failed to find any significant relationships between variables of the family situation and those of the child's asthma. On the other hand, many strong positive relationships were found between extent of family disturbance and behavioral indices of maladjustment in the child, thus confirming the meaningfulness of the family measures. These results led the investigators to question the effect of family variables on asthma itself, as distinguished from the effects on the adjustment of the child with asthma.

The subgroup hypothesis would suggest that the extent of psychological disturbance within a family or a child may be relatively independent of the types of stimulation customarily triggering asthmatic responses. What is hypothesized is an interaction between family variables, severity of asthma, and type of stimulation, that is, family variables may be positively related or unrelated to severity depending upon the types of stimulation customarily triggering asthmatic attacks. It seems possible, therefore, that appropriate subdivision of children in the Dubo study may have led to somewhat different results than were obtained.

Of interest also is a paper by Jacobs, Anderson, Eisman, Muller, and Friedman (1971) questioning the inverse relationship between allergic potential and psychopathology found by Block et al. (1964) among two groups of asthmatic children matched for symptom severity. Jacobs et al. found a very low, nonsignificant positive correlation between an index of biological predisposition (eosinophile reaction to histamine injection) and an index of psychological disturbance. They also failed to find psychological differences between allergic subjects scoring high and low on the biological index. There are several differences between the study by Jacobs et al. and both the present investigation and the one by Block et al. At least two of these may be critical. First, Jacobs's allergic group of 29 college student subjects consisted of 13 with symptoms of asthma and 16 with seasonal hay fever symptoms. Second, no data are provided on symptom severity within the allergic group. Thus, when this group was divided into a high and low biologic reaction group (in order to compare them on the psychological dimension) there was no indication of how well equated these two biologic reaction groups were on either symptom type or symptom severity. The authors' suggestion that biological and psychological variables are best conceived of as independent factors that are neither positively nor negatively correlated is not necessarily inconsistent with the views of Block et al., who tend to speak of reciprocal relationships. Jacobs et al. measured the correlation between these two variables within individuals without regard for symptom severity, the resultant of these two and other factors. It is possible for this correlation to be zero and, at the same time, for an inverse biological–psychological relationship to emerge between groups where symptom severity is held equal in two large, well-matched groups differing only in biologic reactivity.

The same indices suggested for clinical evaluation, i.e., symptom response to separation from the family, perceived precipitants of asthma, and APS scores appear to be the most reliable criteria for the research definition of asthmatic subgroups. Laboratory studies on the experimental induction of asthma represent one promising line of exploration that has not yet involved the identification of subgroups as part of the research strategy. Much of this work is summarized by Purcell, Weiss, and Hahn (1972). Finally, the possibility exists and should be explored that careful description of other psychosomatic disorders, e.g., ulcers, hypertension, will lead to equally fruitful subgroup classifications. If experience with asthma represents any guide, then basing the classification on analyses of the specific events that exacerbate or relieve the particular response involved is likely to be more useful than relying on such general descriptions as type of personality constellation, degree of psychopathology, or quality of interpersonal relationships.

CONCLUDING REMARKS

In the space remaining I should like to comment on two issues that appear to me important to recognize in any serious study of asthma from the psychological point of view. The first concerns the impact of the symptom upon the behavior of the child and his family and the second deals with the impact of problem definition on the behavior of the investigator or clinician.

Impact of the Symptom on the Child and Family

What follows is based largely upon extensive clinical experience rather than careful measurement, but it provides a context that should be understood by any systematic investigators of family relationships, personality, and asthma.

Between attacks, children may regard their symptoms with anxiety and apprehension, or with disgust and embarrassment. They are frequently inhibited by the fear that their symptoms are conspicuous. They may feel different or weaker than others because they cannot keep up with them in physical activity. Persistent feelings of frustration about physical and social deficits are common. A study comparing identification patterns in asthmatic and nonasthmatic boys (Purcell & Clifford, 1966) bears on this question of inadequacy feelings and possible consequences. We found a significant positive relationship between perceived father power and selective attention toward the father (as contrasted with mother) in nonasthmatic boys. This positive relationship is consistent with previous findings (Bandura, Ross, & Ross, 1963; Mussen & Distler, 1959). However, the data also revealed a significant *negative* relationship between these two variables for asthmatic boys. One possible interpretation of these results rests on the clinically based suggestion that severely asthmatic boys who, as a group, have been physically handicapped and dependent, may find inactive, passive fathers less anxiety arousing than more vigorous fathers. Therefore, the preferred male model may be the father who is perceived as less powerful. It is also possible, perhaps even likely, that this observation is not peculiar to asthmatic parent–child relationships but rather is associated with chronic illness.

Resentment and bitterness may develop toward physicians for seeming to promise cures without results. Parents experience so many different schools of approach toward their children's asthma, for example, dietary, the creation of an allergenically controlled environment, psychological, etc., that they tend to become both confused and embittered if these approaches do not work. They make the rounds of physicians in the community, and physicians often understandably react with frustration in seeking to cope with this frequently refractory symptom.

The existence of a child who is asthmatic, particularly if the condition is severe, is often felt as a potent emotional and financial burden by other family members. Parents frequently report a deep sense of guilt for having produced or fostered the development of asthma in a child. Sometimes they point to a genetic mode of transmission; sometimes they believe that bad behaviors on their part have created the symptom. When a patient's symptom is severe enough to warrant constant attention or significant financial drain, the parent may become irritable, resentful, and guilt-ridden. This guilt appears to be one of the antecedents of the commonly observed overprotective maternal attitide toward the asthmatic child, with reciprocal overdependence of the child on the mother.

Not infrequently, overprotective responses are elicited from physicians as well as from parents. The observation of a person in a severe asthmatic attack often arouses marked fear and, subsequent to this, various sorts of restrictions may be urged on the patient by the physician to avoid the anxiety and the responsibility of perhaps having to cope with an episode that can be life threatening.

Impact of the Definition of the Problem

Any chapter dealing with asthma as a psychosomatic problem ought at least to indicate the posture of its author on the definition of "psychosomatic." An excellent paper by Graham (1967) proposes that "psychological" and "physical" refer to different ways of talking about the *same* event, and not to different events. Thus, "mental" and "physical" are regarded as names of different languages, not of different events. Choice of language is governed by convenience, suitability, precision, and personal preference. Quoting Graham, "psychosomatic or psychophysiologic research is the effort to write the dictionary between the two languages" (p. 59).

The observer's view of the term psychosomatic may have important practical implications both for research and clinical practice. Often the "mind" is not believed capable of producing structural or organic changes (how can a thought produce a hole in the duodenum?) although it is held that "mental" influences can produce functional disorders. These assumptions frequently lead to the conclusion that functional disorders are not physical despite the fact that one can easily provide a physical language description of something as traditionally functional as anxiety.

This line of reasoning may also be associated with serious distortion in the evaluation of symptom severity. A frequently acted-on belief appears to be that a somatic symptom induced by psychological provocation cannot really be serious—certainly not as serious as the same symptom induced by physical provocation. For example, the belief that emotionally triggered asthma is "fake asthma" has been found not only among relatives of the patient but also, on occasion, among physicians. The latter situation once led to a patient in the early stages of status asthmaticus (severe, continuous asthma resistant to treatment) being referred for psychotherapy with the physician feeling "it can't really be serious since everybody knows this patient's asthma is all psychic."

In brief, labeling a disorder "psychologicial" can bias the observer (clinician or researcher) against making a vigorous attempt at a physical language description of the somatic processes underlying functional symptoms. This, in turn, may blind one to effective therapeutic procedures that are associated with "physical" descriptions and concepts. Similary, applying the "physical" label to a disorder makes unlikely any serious effort to determine psychological or emotional factors in the etiology or maintenance of the syndrome. Since this chapter was psychologically oriented, those etiologies most appropriately described in biological terms have been relatively neglected.

REFERENCES

Alexander, B. A. Systematic relaxation and flow rates in asthmatic children: Relationship to emotional precipitants and anxiety. *Journal of Psychosomatic Research,* 1972, **16,** 405–410.

Bandura, A., Ross, D., & Ross, S. A. A comparative test of the status envy, social power and secondary reinforcement theories of identificatory learning. *Journal of Abnormal and Social Psychology,* 1963, **67,** 527–534.

Block, J., Jennings, P. H., Harvey, B., & Simpson, E. Interaction between allergic potential and psychopathology in childhood asthma. *Psychosomatic Medicine,* 1964, **26,** 307-320.

Castaneda, A., McCandless, B. R., & Palermo, D. S. The children's form of the manifest anxiety scale. *Child Development,* 1956, **27, 317–326.**

Criep, L. H. *Clinical immunology and allergy.* New York: Grune & Stratton, 1962.

Dubo, S., McLean, J. A., Cheng, A. Y. T., Wright, H. L., Kaufman, P. E., & Sheldon, J. M. A study of relationships between family situations, bronchial asthma and personal adjustment in children. *Journal of Pediatrics,* 1961, **59,** 402–413.

Freeman, E. H., Feingold, B. F., Schlesinger, K., & Gorman, F. J. Psychological variables in allergic disorders: A review. *Psychosomatic Medicine,* 1964, **26,** 543–575.

French, T. M. & Alexander, F. Psychogenic factors in bronchial asthma. *Psychosomatic Medicine Monographs,* 1941, **4,** No. 1.

Gottlieb, P. M. Changing mortality in bronchial asthma. *Journal of the American Medical Association,* 1964, **187,** 276–280.

Graham, D. T. Health, disease, and the mind–body problem: Linguistic parallelism. *Psychosomatic Medicine,* 1967, **24,** 52–71.

Hamburg, D. A. Plasma and corticosteroid plasma levels in naturally occurring psychological stresses. In S. Korey (Ed.), *Ultrastructure and metabolism of the nervous system.* Baltimore: Williams & Wilkins, 1962.

Handlon, J. H., Wadeson, R. W., Fishman, J. R., Sacher, B. J., Hamburg, D. A., & Mason, J. W. Psychological factors lowering plasma 17-hydroxicorticosteroid concentration. *Psychosomatic Medicine,* 1962, **24,** 535–541.

Jacobs, M. A., Anderson, S., Bisman, H. D., Muller, J. J., & Friedman, S. Interaction of psychologic and biologic predisposing factors in allergic disorders. *Psychosomatic Medicine,* 1967, **24,** 572–585.

Miklich, D. R., Chai, C., Purcell, K., Weiss, J. H., & Brady, K. Naturalistic observation of emotions preceding low pulmonary flow rates. *Journal of Allergy and Clinical Immunology,* 1974, **53,** 102. (Abstract of paper presented at meetings of American Academy of Allergy, January, 1974).

Miklich, D. R., Rewey, H. H., Weiss, J. H., & Kolton, S. A preliminary investigation of psychophysiological responses to stress among different subgroups of asthmatic children. *Journal of Psychosomatic Research,* 1973, **17,** 1–8.

Miklich, D. R., Purcell, K., & Weiss, J. H. Practical aspects of the development and use of radio telemetry in behavioral research. *Behavior Research Methods and Instrumentation,* in press.

Mussen, P. & Distler, L. Masculinity, identification, and father–son relationships. *Journal of Abnormal and Social Psychology,* 1959, **52**, 358–362.

Mustacchi, P., Lucia, S. P., & Jassy, L. Bronchial asthma: Patterns of morbidity and mortality in United States. *California Medicine,* 1962, **96**, 196–200.

Neuhaus, P. C. Personality study of asthmatic and cardiac children. *Psychosomatic Medicine,* 1958, **3**, 181–186.

Porter, R. B. & Cattell, R. B. *Handbook for the IPAT children's personality questionnaire.* Champaign, Illinois: Institute for Personality and Ability Testing, 1960.

Proctor, D. F. Physiology of the upper airway. In W. O. Fenn & H. Rahn (Ed.), *Handbook of physiology.* Vol. 1. Baltimore: Waverly Press, Inc., 1964, pp. 309–345.

Purcell, K. Distinctions between subgroups of asthmatic children: Children's perceptions of events associated with asthma. *Pediatrics,* 1963, **31**, 486–494.

Purcell, K. Distinctions between subgroups of asthmatic children: Parental reactions to experimental separations. *Journal of Abnormal Child Psychology,* 1973, 1, 2–15.

Purcell, K., Bernstein, L., & Bukantz, S. C. A preliminary comparison of rapidly remitting and persistently "steroid dependent" asthmatic children. *Psychosomatic Medicine,* 1961, **23**, 305–310.

Purcell, K. & Brady, K. Assessment of interpersonal behavior in natural settings: A research technique and manual. *Final Progress Report MH08415,* 1965, pp. 1–294.

Purcell, K. & Brady, K. Adaptation to the invasion of privacy: Monitoring behavior with a miniature radio transmitter. *Merrill-Palmer Quarterly of Behavior and Development,* 1966, **12**, 242–254.

Purcell, K., Brady, K., Chai, H., Muser, J., Molk, L., Gordon, N., & Means, J. The effect on asthma in children of experimental separation from the family. *Psychosomatic Medicine,* 1969, **31**, 144–164.

Purcell, K. & Clifford, E. Binocular rivalry and the study of identification in asthmatic and nonasthmatic boys. *Journal of Consulting Psychology,* 1966, **30**, 388–394.

Purcell, K. & Metz, J. R. Distinctions between subgroups of asthmatic children: Some parent attitude variables related to age of onset of asthma. *Journal of Psychosomatic Research,* 1962, **6**, 251–258.

Purcell, K., Muser, J., Miklich, D., & Dietiker, K. A comparison of psychologic findings in variously defined asthmatic subgroups. *Journal of Psychosomatic Research,* 1969, **13**, 67–75.

Purcell, K., Turnbull, J. W., Bernstein, L. Distinctions between subgroups of asthmatic children: Psychological test and behavior rating comparisons. *Journal of Psychosomatic Research,* 1962, **6**, 283–291.

Purcell, K., & Weiss, J. Asthma. In C. G. Costello (Ed.), *Symptoms of psychopathology.* New York: Wiley, 1970, pp. 587–623.

Purcell, K., Weiss, J., & Hahn, W. Certain psychosomatic disorders. In B. Wolman (Ed.), *Manual of child psychopathology.* New York: McGraw-Hill, 1972, pp. 706–740.

Rackeman, F. H. & Edwards, M. D. Medical progress: Asthma in children: follow-up study of 688 patients after 20 years. *New England Journal of Medicine,* 1952, **246,** 815–858.

Ratner, B. & Silberman, A. E. Critical analysis of the hereditary concept of allergy. *Journal of Allergy,* 1953, **24,** 371–378.

Reinberg, A., Chata, D., & Sidi, E. Nocturnal asthma attacks and their relationship to the circadian adrenal cycle. *Journal of Allergy,* 1963, **34,** 323–330.

Schiffer, C. G. & Hunt, E. P. *Illness among children.* Washington, D.C.: Children's Bureau, U. S. Dept. of Health & Welfare, 1963.

Schwartz, M. Heredity in bronchial asthma: A clinical and genetic study of 191 asthma probands. *Acta Allergologica,* 1952, **5** (Suppl. 2); 1–288.

Simonsson, B. G., Jacobs, F. M., & Nadel, J. A. Role of autonomic nervous system and the cough reflex in the increased responsiveness of airways in patients with obstructive airway disease. *The Journal of Clinical Investigation,* 1967, **46,** 1812–1818.

Smyth, F. S. Allergy. In B. L. Holt, R. McIntosh, & H. L. Barnett (Eds.), *Pediatrics.* (13th ed.) New York: Appleton-Century, Crofts, 1962.

Zuckerman, M. Reversed scales to control acquiescence response set in the parental attitude research instrument. *Child Development,* 1959, **30,** 523–540.

CHAPTER 4

Minimal Brain Dysfunction and Psychopathology in Children

C. KEITH CONNERS

INTRODUCTION

The concept of minimal brain dysfunction (MBD) has a peculiar place in the medical psychology of children: it is at one and the same time a very widely used label for characterizing children, and one of the most disputed concepts in the field. It is a term used as much by educators as physicians, and among the latter it is often the pediatrician, not the psychiatrist or neurologist, who calls upon this diagnosis.

The reasons for both the wide use and the dispute are reasonably clear. Historically, child psychiatry and the child guidance movement in this country were predominantly influenced by the native American optimism that believes in the perfectibility of the human spirit and has always done so, at least since de Toqueville. This largely humanistic tradition of regarding the child as a malleable product shaped by the benign or malevolent influences of family life, correctable by education, appropriate nurturance and family restructuring, was also strongly influenced in the twentieth century by the ideas of Freud. Those ideas led the search for explanations of child behavior back to the dynamic interplay of the child in the family drama; towards a search for the maternal, paternal, and sibling influences that could account for deviant behavior or developmental arrest; and away from the temperamental, genetic, and organic components of behavior. Despite Freud's original neurological bias, and his early brilliant work on neurological development in children, it was the *environmental* sources of behavior that captured the imagination of the early pioneers in child guidance and child psychiatry partly, one assumes, because of a belief in the mutability of the environment. Other pioneers such as Seguin, Witmer, and Itard also contributed towards a view of child psychiatry that stressed the educability of the child, the role of family life, and the need for a social intervention approach to developmental problems.

There is no question that this historical trend of looking for psychogenic and environmental influences on child development has been a productive and important one. At the same time, another trend of conceptual development has taken place independently and somewhat parallel to the major theme in children's medical psychology. Following the pandemic of von Economo's encephalitis in the 1920s, a syndrome of "post-encephalitic behavior disorder" was described by several workers (Bond & Smith, 1935). This syndrome of hyperactive, impulsive, irritable and explosive behavior came to be described as "organic drivenness," "minimal brain damage," and later, the "Strauss syndrome," reflecting the work of Strauss and his co-workers in identifying apparently "organic" influences in the disordered behavior pattern of a small number of carefully studied children. Subsequent work by Knobloch and Pasamanick (1966) documented an association between prematurity, prenatal, and paranatal complications and certain behavior and learning disorders, with the highest degree of association found between reproductive abnormalities and the hyperactive, disorganized, and confused child.

The logic of these discoveries appears to have proceeded on the assumption that, since organic influences are known to sometimes produce a picture of a hyperkinetic, impulsive child, often having signs of developmental, perceptual, or cognitive dysfunctions, it therefore follows that the recognition of such characteristics may lead one to infer the presence of organic causes or etiology for the disorder. Critics have been quick to point out the error of *post hoc, ergo propter hoc,* but despite the difficulties in documenting brain lesions or gaining other "hard" evidence of brain involvement, the label of "brain dysfunction" or "brain damage" has remained an important and frequently used concept. Several scientific conferences of specialists in the field led to the adoption of the term "minimal brain dysfunction" instead of brain damage, in recognition of the fact that although behavioral deficits are suggestive of brain involvement, definitive evidence of damage at a direct level is usually not available.

Some clinicians such as Blau (1954), after initially believing that the hyperkinetic behavior syndrome was due to brain damage, switched to the belief (in Blau's case, 20 years later), that the syndrome is mainly psychogenic, and that such children actually have an anxiety neurosis that is the result of inadequate superego development.

The use of the concept is further complicated by the complexity of the research findings available. Although a fairly high percentage of hyperactive children* show various signs of neurological involvement, including abnormal

*Throughout this chapter we refer to the "hyperactive" child and the "hyperkinetic child" as interchangeable terms. One should perhaps heed Leo Kanner's etymologic advice not to mix Latin and Greek suffixes (Greek, *kinetikos* = pertaining to motion; Latin, *actio* = motion); and I think

coordination or perception, EEG abnormalities, neurologic soft-signs, pre- or perinatal trauma, disorders of vegetative functions or of major developmental tasks, these characteristics have not shown high associations whenever research has started by sampling these abnormalities, and then trying to find the degree of presence or absence of associated hyperactivity (Werry, 1968). For example, hyperactivity is not a prominent feature of children with brain damage due to fetal anoxia (Graham et al., 1962).

Discovery of brain–behavior relationships is further complicated by the fact that simple quantitative measures of locomotion or energy expenditure are not necessarily reliable indicators of the clinical syndrome as defined by experienced clinicians. Studies have shown that qualitative aspects of motor performance are important, and that it is the lack of goal-oriented behavior, the poor integration of activity, or its brief duration in a goal-oriented sequence, that is characteristic of the child defined as deviant (see, for instance, the excellent study by Pope, 1970).

These considerations have led some authors to view hyperkinesis as a multidimensional disorder, with a variety of distinctive etiologies, only some of which are organic. Bax, an English physician, restricts the term hyperkinetic behavior syndrome in the following way:

> The child with true hyperkinesia has a short attention span and excess motor activity, characteristics which are consistently observed by all adults who come into contact with the child (Bax, 1972).

He separates this relatively uncommon disorder from simple "overactivity," pointing out that in the survey of Rutter et. al of 2000 children on the Isle of Wight, only one child with the "true" syndrome was identified. Instead, he identifies seven main groups of overactive school children: (1) children with psychiatric disturbance, usually neurotic or antisocial; (2) children with specific learning difficulties; (3) children exposed to inappropriate educational tasks; (4) children from social backgrounds inappropriate to the educational system; (5) children whose cultural background is inappropriate to the educational setting; (6) children exposed to inappropriate educational milieu; and (7) children with high drive. Thus, in one sense the hyperactive child is understood as a very uncommon disorder, which, when found, can be assumed to be organic in origin; and it is also understood as a set of more specific syndromes of nonorganic etiology that would apparently become clear with careful clinical examination.

One problem with this approach is that it may be quite difficult to operation-

---

it preferable to distinguish between hyperactivity as a symptom, and the *hyperkinetic syndrome;* which should have a much more precise meaning. For the description of the latter, the reader is referred to Laufer's original description (Laufer, Denhoff, & Solomons, 1957) and to the excellent review chapter by Wender and Eisenberg (1974).

alize the concept if the behavior must be consistently observed by all adults coming into contact with the child. Klein and Klein (1974) showed that a trained social worker could not reliably identify children from maternal interview as hyperkinetic even though they were plainly hyperactive in school and in the clinic. As they say, "Such findings should engender a relatively high degree of scepticism concerning negative maternal reports regarding hyperactivity at home." Moreover, there is no obvious logical reason why situational specificity should not be considered in defining the syndrome, since it is a truism of behavioral analysis that the organism behaves differently in different stimulus environments. This would seem to hold true whether direct brain dysfunction is demonstrable or not, so that trans-situational hyperactivity seems like an unnecessarily rigid and restrictive requirement, more appropriate to a definition of *severity,* rather than to understanding of etiology.

Despite the justified criticisms of over inclusive or vague definition of the syndrome, failure to prove organic etiology unequivocally, logical errors in "organicizing" behavior, the multidimensional nature of the behavior patterns and their origins, the concept of minimal brain dysfunction has continued to have an appeal, and an apparently increasingly ubiquitous presence, either through increased prevalence of the disorder or because of some powerful social and quasiscientific reasons to maintain the concept.

I believe that the fundamental reason for the persistence of MBD as a diagnostic or scientific concept has to do with the heuristic value on the one hand, and the implied command to act in a certain way, on the other. Let me explain: As long as deviant behavior patterns were generally thought of as largely or simply the end result of learned patterns acquired in the child's family, the social and behavioral scientist usefully directed his attention to the relevant variables in those domains, and reaped a fair harvest of knowledge regarding the antecedents of behavioral disorders in children, as well as antecedents of normal child development. The role of attachment, nurturing, identification, imitation, cognitive stimulation, and many such factors in child development, both normal and abnormal, are now well accepted.

But once it is assumed that some exogenous or genetic factor might interfere with brain function, and this defect in turn leads to the pattern of disordered, poorly integrated, impulsive, and ill-modulated behavior characteristic of the "MBD child," entirely different variables are investigated. This point can be illustrated by a study that related serum lead levels to hyperactivity. Hyperkinetic children who had a known or probable basis for the disorder (e.g., extremely low birth weight), did not differ from controls in lead levels, whereas the "pure" cases with no assignable cause showed significantly higher levels of serum lead (David et al., 1972). The authors of this study comment that

Hyperactivity is a symptomatic state, not a disease. Being able to segregate a group of such children where the aetiology is known (e.g., due to lead) would be extremely helpful and might be useful in further research of the hyperactive child syndrome.

Such studies in turn lead to biochemical investigations of mechanism having much wider implications for understanding of the mechanism of the disorder. For example, an animal model of lead-induced hyperactivity has been developed to test the hypothesis that the immediate cause of the hyperactivity is the tendency of lead to alter the ratio of central dopamine to epinephrine (Sauerhoff & Michaelson, 1973). Further examples of the heuristic value of the concept of MBD will be discussed later in this chapter.

Another basic reason for the survival and growth of the MBD concept is its implied suggestion of a therapeutic approach different from the conventional approaches, which have largely been based upon a psychogenic formulation of the disorders being treated. It seems reasonably clear that physicians, psychiatrists, and especially educators have become disenchanted with the slow progress achieved over the past 100 years in remediation and therapeutic intervention with this intractable group of children by the conventional child guidance, psychotherapy-oriented team approach. By formulating the problem in terms of brain function, the clinician or educator may feel more comfortable with somatic therapies (such as pharmacotherapy), and may be more inclined to explore perceptual or motor correlates and methods of training the brain to function more normally (as in the many techniques descended from the Strauss and Lehtinen studies). In this sense, the MBD concept is also heuristic with regard to new methods of treatment. The need for such methods is clearly illustrated by the data from Table 1: The results of brief treatment with several methods were compared, including brief psychotherapy, tranquilizing drugs, placebos, and brief guidance and counselling. In these studies the psychiatrists rated the children's improvements by a global rating method. Interestingly and disappointingly, none of the treatments produced significiant advantages over other treatments. However, as the table illustrates, there is a significant difference in the distribution of improvement among the neurotic and hyperkinetic children, with the latter being quite refractory to improvement compared to neurotic children, two-thirds of whom improve regardless of the form of therapy. Data such as these are persuasive reasons for shifting to alternative modes of treatment (including different types of drugs).

Whether such alternative therapeutic methods are in fact more desirable from the standpoint of social utility, ethics, degree of cost, and amount of benefit are complex issues still to be decided. The point being made here, however, is simply that the very formulation of the problem in terms of brain dysfunction is a method for shifting the focus of research and clinical practice. At any one point in time such a concept as MBD may be found to be wanting in terms of empirical justification or conceptual clarity, but its use has a

Table 1.   Results of Brief Treatment

Diagnosis	Improvement		Total
	Marked	Mild or None	
Neurotic	48	23	71
Hyperkinetic	37	96	133
Total	85	119	204

$p < 0.001$.

powerful social impetus in redirecting the energy and resources expended in the search for understanding of basic mechanisms and new forms of therapy. Whether such a redirection is ultimately successful in the production of new knowledge, or has a pernicious effect in distracting one from more socially relevant variables, the fact of the MBD concept as a heuristic force seems undeniable, and is perhaps its best raison d'etre.

MINIMAL BRAIN DYSFUNCTION AND SITUATIONAL STRESS RESPONSE

We have seen that the argument is sometimes raised that, since hyperactivity may appear in some situations and not in others, a prima facie case is made against a biological basis for the disorder. The most common disclaimer in this respect comes from parents who find the child acceptable at home, but a terror in school, and therefore assume that something is wrong with the school, or that the child's problems are simply educational in nature, requiring restructuring of the educational setting. Apart from the fact of differing parental thresholds of tolerance for disorganized behavior, three significant differences exist between home and school that could conceivably account for the difference in behavior.

First, there is the element of social aggregation or social stimulation. As is well known in animal studies, physiological effects, including the threshold for fatal response to drugs, aggression, tolerance for extremes of temperature, and other behaviors, are profoundly influenced by the density of social aggregation in the animal living environment. Conceivably, similar social aggregation effects could affect a child with brain dysfunction in a deleterious way, either through the excess of stimulation over the child's capacity for regulating input, or through some fundamental releasing mechanism that acts to weaken inhibitory controls.

Second, in school there are usually increased cognitive demands, including requirements of more rapid perceptual and discrimination response. Such demands could interact with built-in limits on "channel capacity" in children with central processing abnormalities, or in children who have a delay in maturation of the central processing systems. This interaction between information load and the commonly found "distractibility" of the hyperkinetic child can be illustrated by a study I conducted some years ago, using children diagnosed as hyperactive by a child psychiatrist on the basis of history and clinical examination.

The children were provided with a search task in which they had to cross out a "small red" target in a display that had orthogonal combinations of shape, size, color, and solidity to give either a two-, three-, or four-bit information load.* The task was performed twice, once under distracting noise and once without noise, with half the subjects getting noise first, and half no-noise conditions first. The design of the study is shown in Figure 1.

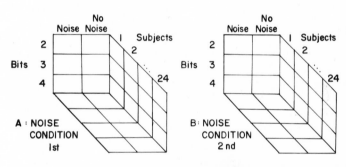

Ss received all 6 conditions (two noise x three bits) with order of bits randomized independently for each S. One group (N = 24) received noise 1st., the other group received no-noise 1st.

Figure 1.   Experimental design for study of information processing under distraction.

The results of the study are shown in Figure 2. The top half of the figure shows the number of errors made for 2, 3, or 4 bits of information. It appears

*In information theory, a unit of information is called a bit, which is short for "binary digit." If a stimulus reduces one's uncertainty it is said to carry information; if it reduces one's uncertainty by dividing the alternatives in half, as for example when one tries to guess which square on the chess board I am thinking of, and you ask if the square is on the left half, the amount of information is said to be one bit. The number of bits is the log to the base 2, of the number of alternatives.

that the effect of the distraction becomes more crucial as the information load in the stimulus goes up. Therefore, one might well assume that a distractible child will often show his disability only under conditions of increased information load. In this experiment, the children are asked to make a simple perceptual discrimination, and in each case the number of items in the display, and the number of correct target items remains constant, with only the amount of information in the display varying between tasks. The effect of the "distraction" only becomes apparent at the higher information levels—an effect not unexpected since the distraction consisted of the experimenter saying "red, large, solid, blue, etc." while the child was actively searching for the small red item.

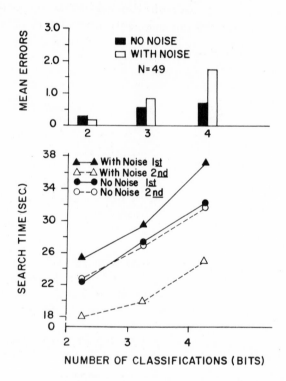

Figure 2.   Results of study showing interaction of distracting "noise" upon errors and search time in information processing task. As more information is added to the task, the children show more sensitivity to the disruptive influence of noise.

An even more important lesson can be drawn from this study. The lower set of curves in Figure 2 shows that the effect of the distraction depends upon degree of prior practice with the task. If the children got "noise" first, their search time was quite slow compared to the second time they performed the tasks without noise. When no noise was given it did not make any difference whether they had prior practice with the task. Thus, the distraction effect is dependent upon degree of practice which should affect the rate at which the information can be handled, and the noise may actually *facilitate* performance, as it appeared to do here, if the task had been previously practiced. These results suggest that the child with brain dysfunction may require *stimulation* rather than reduced distraction under certain conditions, especially under conditions where the task is either well practiced or overlearned. The role of "stimulus seeking" in hyperactivity and the implied defect in the central and peripheral nervous systems of these children will be discussed in later sections of this chapter.

Further analysis of this study was carried out by giving each subject a score, representing the extent to which his performance was impaired by the distracting noise. This score was found to be related to the success with which the children could accurately deal with the Muller-Lyer illusion, the horizontal-vertical illusion, and a test in which colors must be read from a distracting background consisting of color names in conflict with the colors to be identified (e.g. the color "red" might be painted over the *word* "blue," causing the subject to respond inaccurately and/or more slowly). Thus, the distractibility of these children—as measured by the slowing of information processing under distraction—significantly affects the perceptual accuracy or the ability to give a verdical perceptual judgment. As we have seen, this distractibility may only become apparent where the rate (amount of information to be processed in unit time) of environmental demand is high, as in the school situation.

A similar interaction between rate of information demand and simple visual discriminations in hyperkinetic children was shown in a study comparing the effects of dextroamphetamine and placebo (Conners, 1966). Figure 3 shows that the effect of the drug in reducing discrimination errors (in a task involving size discrimination) depended upon the rate (or degree of stress as this was interpreted) at which the discriminations had to be made. Again, the point to be made with these data is that the pathology of the child may become apparent only under certain environmental conditions, and the role of treatments such as pharmacotherapy may depend upon the nature of the environmental demands placed upon the child. Obviously, such data have found profound implications for the question of the circumstances under which medications might be useful or necessary. It might be better to arrange for the child to have fewer distractions, low information rate, and less stress than to give him a psychotropic drug. On the other hand, these changes may not be realistic, or the thresholds in the child so low, that no other alternative is satisfactory. In most cases the titration of one variable against the other is appropriate, and a simple-minded answer to the question, "Are drugs good for the child?" is unwise and unwarranted. The main point to be made in this section is that MBD as a concept is not vitiated simply because the environ-

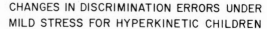

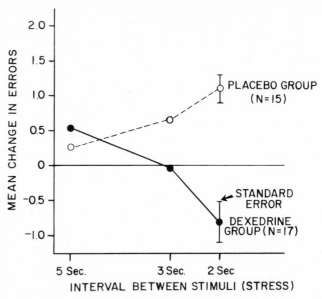

Figure 3. Discrimination performance of hyperkinetic children treated with dextroamphetamine or placebo. The figure shows the increase in errors in the placebo group and the decrease in the drug group as the stress of the task is increased. Children had to judge which of six circles was the largest. Drug-treated children show improved performance under stress compared to placebo-treated children.

ment elicits the pathological behavior in some circumstances and not others.

A third factor in the difference between home and school that might account for apparently different behavior in the two settings, is the degree of structure of the situation which is required, and the extent to which lapses in attention penalize the child. As Douglas and co-workers have shown (Douglas, 1974), hyperkinetic children do more poorly on an experimenter-paced task than a subject-paced vigilance task. School is much more likely than home to have a "fixed schedule" of activity, and to penalize the child for not keeping time with the external authority (teacher). Many times, educational intervention with such children takes the form of providing a freer atmosphere of subject-paced activity. On the other hand, it may sometimes be necessary to have *more* structure in the classroom, precisely because the MBD child loses his way so readily.

The role of environmental structure in revealing disorders of brain function is a special case of the general problem of the role of attentional and focusing mechanisms in guiding the child's social and cognitive processing. Several investigators have noted that a key defect in hyperactive and MBD children seems to be their inability to maintain a focus of attention. The MBD child's problems with attention are notorious, but the concept itself is a difficult one to operationalize, and its relation to other concepts such as "arousal" are complex. Nevertheless, the somewhat vague clinical notion that the MBD child typically has a "short attention span" leads us to ask the question of whether there is any evidence for a disorder of brain mechanisms that control attention in the child with MBD.

One recent approach to this problem has been to combine behavioral and direct brain recording methods through the use of the averaging computer to obtain "cortical evoked responses."

Unfortunately, as most people are aware, there are many technical and conceptual ambiguities in this method, so that in one sense the inquiry may be but another example of "trying to correlate the mysterious with the unknown."

In this method, electrodes are attached to the scalp and electrical potentials are amplified by conventional methods. Repeated sensory stimulation is time-locked to a computor averager, which stores the response following each stimulus. The pattern of response to the very small electrical potentials can then be recovered since the signal-to-noise ratio improves as a function of the number of trials. In effect, the random "noise" averages out, while the signal components summate. The later components of this response, between 200 and 300 milliseconds, have a number of important behavioral correlates, especially to the information value of the stimulus and the subject's attentional state.

In previous studies we found that the stimulant drugs enhance these late components of the ER, and latencies were reduced. However, the effects were not very large and were not predictive of the degree of clinical drug response. In a second study, we hypothesized that the drug effect might be more noticeable if the subjects' attention was manipulated. By presenting both auditory and visual stimuli intermittently, and instructing the subject to attend to one or the other modality (and ensuring that he did so by forcing him to make a discrimination in the selected modality), we were able to show that the drugs had a highly significant effect on amplitudes *when the subject was attending to that modality.* Moreover, we found that the two stimulants we were comparing— dextroamphetamine and magnesium pemoline—had somewhat different effects: amphetamine increased amplitudes under the attention condition, but pemoline increased amplitudes under attention, and decreased amplitudes in the nonattending condition (Conners, 1974).

Although there is some disagreement in the literature, the late component we referred to is often described as a 'nonspecific" ER component since it is evoked by most sensory modalities and has its largest amplitude at the vertex rather than at the primary sensory receiving areas. This so-called "vertex potential" clearly appears to be of cerebral origin, and undergoes marked changes as a function of the uncertainty or information value of the stimulus. To further test the notion that the effect of the stimulant drugs on hyperkinetic children is an effect related to an enhancement of selective attention, or increased control under conditions of multiple sensory stimulation, we decided to examine the effects of drugs on the vertex potential in the following manner.

The children had a single electrode attached to the vertex, with a reference to the right mastoid. A light flash and a brief tone burst were presented in a random sequence, with one-third of the trials having a simultaneous onset of both stimuli. Thus, there were three stimuli: light (L), sound (S), and a combined light and sound (L + S). We predicted that the vertex response would be larger to the combined stimuli, either as a result of simple summation of neuronal ensembles activated at the same time, or because of the heightened arousal produced by the stimuli in combination.

We also predicted that this amplification process would be more effective under the influence of stimulant medication. We predicted that even though the drugs might have a minimal effect on the light or sound vertex response, the effect on the combined response would be significant. In effect, we are predicting that the drugs will enhance the capability of the subject for dealing with simultaneous stimuli, an effect that should show up as an increased vertex potential relative to the nondrug state, and irrespective of whether the individual stimuli produce increased amplitudes under the drug state.

One hundred and twenty-eight signals were averaged for each of the three stimulus conditions. The subjects were given no instructions, other than to sit quietly. The light was delivered with eyes closed by a photostimulator, and the tone was a clipped sine wave delivered through a loudspeaker by an audio generator. The subjects were 18 children being studied in a double-blind trial of methylphenidate, magnesium pemoline, and placebo over an 8-week period. ERs were obtained prior to, and on the last day of the treatment period. Drug dosage was increased on a fixed schedule for the first 4 weeks and maintained at the optimum level for the last 4 weeks.

In every case, the combined stimuli evoked a larger (and usually more clearly defined) vertex response than either of the two single stimuli. Interestingly, the combined response sometimes appeared to "mimic" the visual response, and sometimes the auditory, and sometimes both, as though one modality was preferred or attended to more regularly by the subject. Figures 4 and 5 show examples of contrasting responses. The small number of subjects precludes examining clinical response by these interesting qualitative variations, but the results immediately suggest an objective method for identifying a preferred modality that may have relevance to the child's learning style.

The changes produced by the drugs as compared with placebo are shown in Figure 6. There is no significant change in either the single auditory or visual response between drug and placebo. However, there is a significant increase

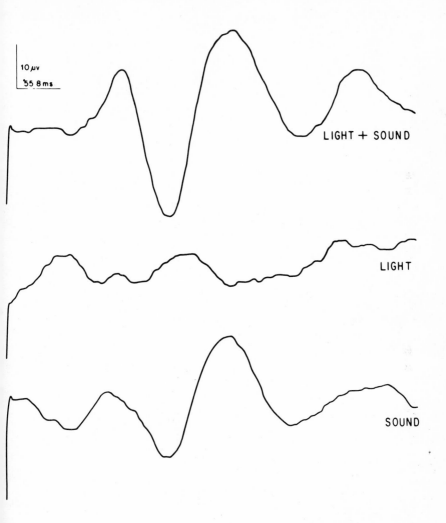

Figure 4. Visual evoked responses elicited by light, sound, or simultaneous light and sound. The combined stimulus effect is largely due to the sound.

in the amplitude of the vertex potential for the *combined* stimuli for the drug-treated subjects.

Apparently, then, the stimulant drugs increase the cortical response to multiple stimuli above and beyond the increases produced in the individual stimuli by themselves. We are not sure what these increases mean, but in line

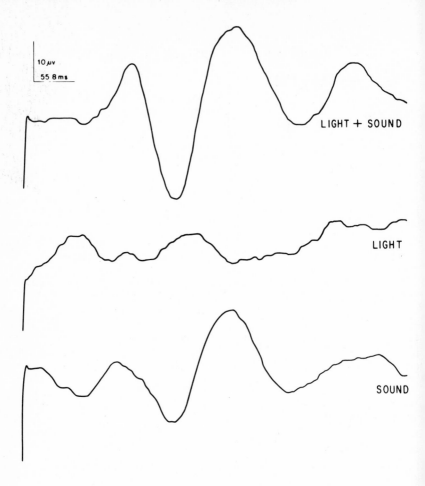

Figure 5. Visual evoked responses elicited by light, sound, or simultaneous light and sound. The combined stimulus effect is largely due to the light.

with our hypothesis we tend to believe that the major effect of the drugs is to increase the capacity of the subject to maintain an alert, active, and controlled state while being subjected to multiple stimuli from the environment. Our cortical evoked response findings of increased activation under multiple sensory stimulation in the medication condition may mean that the reserve of

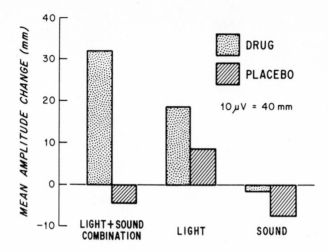

Figure 6.   Effect of stimulant drugs on visual evoked response amplitude for three conditions of stimulation. Changes are expressed in millimeters from proportional X–Y plots.

arousal needed to cope with such stimuli is increased, thus allowing accurate information processing without concomitant reduction of attention to an ongoing task.

Needless to say, we are convinced that within the sample studied here, there is great heterogeneity at several levels. More detailed analysis may show that some of the children respond to drug treatment by showing greater selective attention to one modality over the other, while others show attention to both or neither.Nevertheless, the findings of increased vertex arousal might be an important clue for the detection of those "drug-specific" hyperkinetic children for whom this treatment is rationally justified.

HETEROGENEITY AND THE PROBLEM OF DIAGNOSIS

Much of the experimental work with MBD children, especially those labeled as hyperkinetic, has involved comparisons of MBD children with either normals or other patient groups. This is a standard method in medicine for elucidating the phenomenology, pathophysiology, response to treatment, natural history, and prognosis of a disease state. As a minimum requirement for such investigations one must have operational criteria for identifying the target patient group, and be able precisely to specify the characteristics that define the group as contrasted with normal persons or other controls.

It is not necessary that the differentiating characteristic be a single property such as the presence of a certain virus or pathogen; there may be a group of characteristics that cluster together, either uniformly so that the same set of characteristics is always found with the disorder, or such that a pool of characteristics is drawn upon, even though any two individuals may never show exactly the identical set of traits. These approaches, involving a fixed set or variable set define a monothetic or polythetic class, respectively, as these terms are used in taxonomic systems in biology (Sokal, 1974). MBD would appear to satisfy the requirements for a polythetic class since it is generally impossible to point to a single characteristic (such as short attention span), nor do all MBD children have the same set of "cardinal" traits. There is no single historical incident or pattern that unequivocally leads to the diagnosis, and no defining pathological score or test (such as EEG) that can be used in all cases. These facts have led some workers to be sceptical of the concept and to doubt its use. However, I believe that this is characteristic of all heuristically valuable concepts in the early stages of scientific development, and what is required is a plan and methods to make advances in refining the concept.

One is in a peculiar "bootstrap" position in the early phases of investigation: It is impossible to select patients with a uniform picture because of the absence of unequivocal markers for the disorder; and without some degree of homogeneity of the patient population, one will be unable to discover any single or unique factors that dispose to brain dysfunction. This point has been previously illustrated by the findings with regard to lead and hyperactivity. The hyperactive children as a group do not differ from controls; it is only when one is able to subdivide them that a group emerges that has lead as a clear antecedent of the disorder.

That the MBD group is *physiologically* heterogeneous is an important statement, for it is upon this basis that ultimate justification for somatic therapies may have to rest, given the ethical and safety factors involved in drug therapy with children. One hypothesis that has emerged from recent work is that some MBD children are autonomically *under*aroused (Satterfield et al., 1974). Satterfield and co-workers have found evidence to suggest that in tasks demanding attention, the MBD child characteristically has a lower level of skin conductance and also shows less power in the alpha range of the EEG spectrum. Those children who improve with stimulants show increased autonomic and central arousal, suggesting that the behavioral state of overactivity may reflect a nervous system state of weakened control (underarousal). To explore the possibility that some children labelled as MBD are in fact distinctive in their pattern of autonomic arousal, a recent study will be described in detail. This study illustrates the issues of heterogeneity of the MBD population, and leads to new empirical support for the emerging hypothesis of a defect in autonomic-central integration and homeostasis in MBD children.*

The aims of this investigation were to explore the possibility of systematic abnormalities of the autonomic nervous system in hyperkinetic children, as evidenced by resting levels and by the course of response to stimuli, and to relate autonomic differences to differences in clinical features of such children.

The experimental subjects were 50 children between the ages of 6 and 12 years, referred by local schools or pediatricians because of a problem of overactivity, and inattentiveness. Questionnaires filled out by teachers and parents were required to show hyperkinetic behavior in both areas for the child to be accepted.

During the child's initial evaluation, psychometric testing was performed, a full history obtained, and psychiatric and neurological examinations were carried out. On the basis of this evaluation, and of an interdisciplinary conference, a number of these children were designated as "acceptable" for a drug study; that is to say that they all received a diagnosis of hyperkinesis due to minimal brain dysfunction, were of IQ more than 80, were free of sensory or major neurological defect or of current physical illness, and were judged not to be suffering from a degree of family psychopathology sufficient to account for their deviations of behavior. Of the 50 children here considered, 31 met these conditions and are described as the "hyperkinetic" group. The remaining 19, the "rejected" group, formed a more heterogeneous set of children; the most common diagnosis among them was that of neurotic reaction.

The control children were 18 children free of known physical or mental illness. Nine were matched by teachers as being similar in age, sex, and grade level to a child undergoing evaluation; ten were the unaffected siblings of children undergoing evaluation. One further "normal" child was seen; but as he proved to have considerable reading difficulties, and as he had bizarre autonomic recordings (probably related to the continuous steroid medication required by his severe asthma), he was rejected from the control group.

Methods

At the same time as the initial evaluation, recordings of skin resistance and finger pulse volume were made. The examiner was blind as to whether the child was a patient or a control; and the polygraph measures were scored only later. These results did not, therefore, affect the diagnostic assessment of the child.

The child sat in a semireclining chair in a blandly furnished sound-attenuated room with normal illumination. The experimenter had previously developed rapport when the child had briefly been shown the testing room. He was reassured that nothing unpleasant would happen. The apparatus was in

*The study reported here was done in my laboratory by Eric Taylor, M.D. Results and analyses described here have not yet been published and are subject to revision for scientific journal presentation.

a separate room; a one-way mirror divided the two.

White noise at approximately 30 dB was presented through a loudspeaker 6 feet from the subject. The temperature of the room was maintained between 72°F and 74.5°F, and the humidity between 10% and 30%.

Skin resistance was recorded via two Beckman silver/silver chloride electrodes, with a diameter of 4 mm. They were attached to the index and ring fingers of the left hand, on the palmar surface of the distal phalanges; if, however, there were abrasions of the skin in that area they were attached to the middle phalanx. The skin was previously washed with acetone and dried; Offner electrode paste was used to make contact between skin and electrodes. A constant current of 5 microamps was passed through the electrodes and the resultant voltage was recorded by a polygraph. From this was calculated the resistance and hence the conductance, the electrode on the index finger being the active electrode.

The finger pulse volume was measured by a photelectric plethysmograph. It was attached to the distal phalanx of the little finger of the left hand; the left arm was supported on the chair arm at approximately the level of the heart and the left hand rested gently, but without restraint, on a supporting plastic cradle. An opaque cloth, supported above the hand, warded off incident light. The voltage output of the transducer was recorded by a separate chanel of the polygraph.

Figure 7 is a reproduction of such a record, and shows the fall in skin resistance and diminution in finger pulse volume following an auditory stimulus.

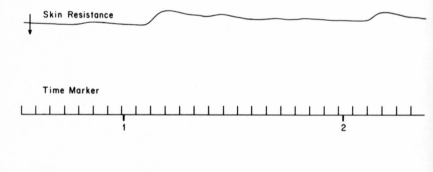

Figure 7. Polygraph record showing changes in skin resistance, and vasoconstrictive response of finger plethysmograph following stimulation by a 100 msec tone (noted on time marker at 1 and 2).

Scoring of records was done manually, but in ignorance of whose record was being scored. During a resting period skin conductance was measured every 30 seconds. A *nonspecific galvanic skin response* (GSR) during a period of rest was defined as a fall in resistance of more than 3.3% of the baseline resistance, followed by a return to the original resistance. A relative measure is preferable to an absolute one (such as "a change of > 800 ohms") in being less dependent on the level of the baseline; this particular level was chosen since at the lowest baseline resistance levels (approximately 30,000 ohms) a change of 1000 ohms was judged to be the minimum level that could in all subjects be distinguished from background noise. In subjects with higher resistance levels a proportionately greater change is required to count as a GSR. Different criteria for a GSR would, of course, effect the results. Here, the nonspecific GSRs were expressed as their frequency per minute.

The latency of a GSR to a specific stimulus was defined as the time in seconds between the onset of the stimulus and the beginning of the response, where a response was any fall of resistance occurring between 0.5 and 4.5 seconds after the onset of the stimulus.

The amplitude of a GSR to a specific stimulus was defined as the difference between the conductance level at the start of the response and the conductance level at the peak of the response; a response here was any fall of resistance between 0.5 and 4.5 seconds after onset of the response. The fact that changes in conductance were used makes some allowance for the size of the initial resistance;

$$\text{If } R_1 = \text{initial resistance}$$
$$R_2 = \text{resistance at peak of response,}$$

then evidently
$$\frac{1}{R_1} - \frac{1}{R_2} = \frac{R_2 - R_1}{R_1 R_2}.$$

The finger pulse volume (FPV) was measured as the distance between peak and trough on the rising part of the waveform. Again, a measure taking baseline into account is necessary and an objective measure was preferred.

The mean of the first three pulses following a stimulus was therefore found, as was the mean of the next three. The differences between these means, weighted for the size of the first three pulses, was taken as an index of the response to a stimulus, i.e.

FPV response =

$$\frac{\text{Mean (Pulse}_1 + \text{Pulse}_2 + \text{Pulse}_3) - \text{Mean (Pulse}_4 + \text{Pulse}_5 + \text{Pulse}_6)}{\text{Mean (Pulse}_1 + \text{Pulse}_2 + \text{Pulse}_3)}$$

No latency measure was therefore appropriate.

Movement artifacts naturally present difficulties in such a group of children.

The electrodermal measures proved happily robust; movement artifacts were few and readily distinguishable from physiological responses. This was not so, however, in pilot trials with larger electrodes; the rather small electrodes were therefore used although it is recognized that they lead to the use of an undesirably high current density.

FPV measures proved practical when the child was exhorted to refrain from major changes of posture. The child was watched through a one-way mirror and, when any major movements of the arm or any major changes in posture occurred during the response to a stimulus, that response was discarded from the analysis. In all, 17 responses in different children had to be discarded, and of these, six children were in the hyperkinetic group, four were in the "rejected" group, and one was a control. The numbers of subjects are therefore diminished in some parts of the analysis.

Procedure

After 5 minutes of general conversation with the child to allay excess apprehension and to allow stabilization of the electrodes, the experimenter left the room after warning the child that in 5 minutes he would hear some tones and should merely listen to them.

Resting levels of conductance and frequency of nonspecific GSR were then recorded over 5 minutes.

Six auditory stimuli were then presented at 15-second intervals. Each tone lasted for 100 msecs and was of approximately 80 dB; it was played through a loudspeaker directly (4 feet) above the child's head. For half the children (chosen randomly) the pitch of the tone was 750 cps; for the other half it was at 1000 cps.

These first six stimuli are described as Block 1.

In Block 2, six further stimuli were played in an identical way, except that those children who had heard high tones in Block 1 now heard low tones, and vice versa.

Electrodermal and FPV changes to each stimulus were measured as described above; each stimulus caused a mark on the polygraph chart to facilitate later scoring.

After the course of habituation had been followed in this way, the experimenter reentered the room and placed a telegraph key on the right arm of the chair. The children were instructed to press for one tone (the "positive" tone) and to withold any response for the other (the "negative" tone). Whether the high or low tone was positive for a given child was determined randomly, and so there are four possible stimulus presentation groups:

1. High tone first in habituation; high tone positive.
2. High tone first in habituation; low tone positive.
3. Low tone first in habituation; high tone positive.
4. Low tone first in habituation; low tone positive.

(Since the inhibition of overt responses appears to be so fundamental a difficulty of hyperkinetic children, it was expected that a greater autonomic response might accompany the successful inhibition of an overt response, as in Jones's concept of the "internalization" of reactions to different stimuli; and further that the overt response and the autonomic response might vary differently in normal children and in hyperkinetics).

After practice on six stimuli, after which time nearly all children were successful in the discrimination, the experimenter again left the child and ten stimuli were presented at 15-second invervals. Five high and five low stimuli were presented in a fixed but unpredictable order. Mechanical counters recorded numbers of correct key responses and of total key responses; a reaction time clock was started by each positive stimulus and stopped by each correct response. Autonomic responses were again measured.

After recording resting levels for a further 60 seconds, the child was released, thanked, and given a small prize. His usual reaction had been one of boredom and fidgetiness. The failure of a few children to complete all parts of the experiment deserves explanation:

1.   Three children had a hearing loss of more than 30 dB in the appropriate frequency range; although their resting levels were measured, it seemed best to exclude them from consideration of reactions to auditory stimuli.

2.   The absence of some data due to movement and so on has already been mentioned. In the majority of analyses to be described, the key variables are means of several readings, and the absence of a single reading probably has little effect.

3.   The 50 patients described come from a population of 62 evaluated at the clinic over the period of this study. Four children proved to be intellectually retarded, and they are not further considered since the subject population for this study was intended to be that of the intellectually normally hyperkinetic child. Six children attended at times when the rigors of the New England climate made the test of skin variables of little value. One child (who had a specific fear of needles and of doctors) was frightened by the experimental situation and was not pressed into it. One child was unfortunately omitted from testing for logistic reasons.

Results

Resting Autonomic Levels

Very little evidence could be found to support the notion that the resting levels of GSR conductance were different among controls, patients, and rejected subjects. There was a slight trend for patients to have more "nonspecific GSRs," that is activation responses occurring in the absence of stimuli, but this trend was slight.

It is only when some subdivision of the patient groups is made on clinical grounds that the picture becomes clearer. First, we may note that the psychiatrist rated the children on degree of anxiety, with zero indicating essentially normal, one being moderate anxiety, and two being marked anxiety. The median skin conductance for these three patient groups are as follows:

Anxiety: 0   1   2
Median Conductance: 13.2   21.8   25.8 (μmhos)

Each of these paired differences, as well as the overall difference among groups, is statistically significant, showing that the children with higher anxiety react with higher autonomic response levels as defined by skin conductance.

Now if one asks the question of how these responses are related to neurological status, one finds no overall relationship with the patient group as a whole. However, when children who are rated as anxious are excluded, a clear relationship with neurological status appears:

Neurological Exam
Normal   Abnormal
Conductance   17.7 μmhos   11.0 μmhos

This difference is statistically significant, and shows that the neurologically abnormal children are significantly *less* aroused than those who have normal neurological examinations, a finding entirely consonant with the recent findings of Satterfield et al. It is important to note, however, that such a relationship only emerges when the putative "hyperkinetic" group is subdivided into a more homogeneous population.

This point is further illustrated by a comparison in which the children are divided in terms of whether their CNS history is normal or abnormal:

CNS History:	Normal	Dubious	Abnormal
Conductance (μmhos)	17.8	13.5	10.2

The difference among these groups is highly significant ($p < .01$), with only the comparison between normal and dubious not significant. Indeed, there is no overlap at all in scores between those with a normal history (lowest value 15.68 μmhos), and those with an abnormal history (highest value 13.63 μmhos)—a result that suggests the test might be useful as a diagnostic tool.

Habituation

There is actually much more reason to be interested in the responsiveness of the nervous system than its resting level; in particular, it is of interest to look at what happens to the nervous system when it is repeatedly stimulated over time. Typically the organism will tend to "habituate," which is the simplest form of adaptation and learning. This is usually shown by a gradual or sudden decrease in the responsiveness to stimulation over time, especially if the stimuli have no appetitive consequences for the organism. That is, unless there is some "pay off" in terms of reward or punishment, it is adaptive for the organism in most circumstances to cease to respond with "attention" in the form of nervous reaction or orienting to the stimuli. Such changes are in fact a reasonable way for looking at failures of central or autonomic adaptation to innocuous stimuli. At one level such tests represent a good operational definition of "distractibility," for if the organism continues to respond to a variety of external, basically innocuous stimuli, it will have any attempts at learning or goal-directed behavior interfered with. Or if its rate of adaptation is significantly faster or slower than normal, the organism may have difficulty in learning to ignore or to attend to relevant cues in the environment.

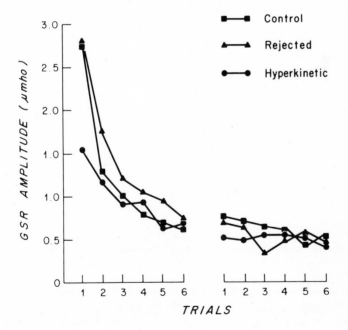

Figure 8. Galvanic skin response amplitude changes with repeated stimulation in hyperkinetic children, matched controls, and clinic patients rejected from the study.

Figure 8 shows the amplitude of the GSR over the six successive trials in each block; and it can be seen that the trend is for hyperkinetic subjects to be *less* responsive initially and *less* rapid in habituation (it might appear that the differences are entirely due to the difference in initial level; but this has been adjusted for statistically by analysis of covariance methods). The same relationships hold when the habituation responses are adjusted for resting GSR levels as well. The differences among hyperkinetics and controls is clearly seen in Figures 9 and 10, which present the data with the first three and the second three trials of each block averaged together—a method that gives greater stability and is less subject to missing data or unreliability of any given trial.

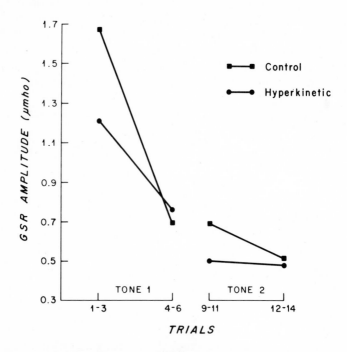

Figure 9. Galvanic skin response amplitude changes for hyperkinetic and control children illustrating the lowered responsiveness of the hyperkinetics.

The *latency* or speed of the GSR response does not appear to differ among the groups, although the trend is usually for the hyperkinetics to respond more slowly, and progressively more so as the experiment proceeds.

A quite similar finding with respect to finger pulse volume can be demonstrated. This measure reflects the degree of vasoconstriction in the finger following stimulation, a purely sympathetic nervous system response, and

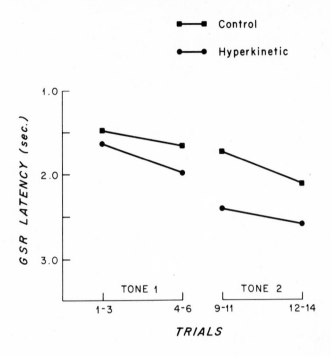

Figure 10.   GSR latency changes of hyperkinetic and control children showing lower responsiveness of hyperkinetics (slower responses).

therefore an important measure of "activation" or arousal response. Figure 11 shows the results with the first three trials of each block averaged together. The control children tend to have a much larger percentage drop in their responsiveness over time than the hyperkinetics, even when the initial differences in response level are taken into account.

Finally, one may ask what happens when the child must discriminate two signals, and respond to one and *inhibit* the other. This is a much more life-like situation for our subjects, and in our opinion, reveals one of the crucial differences between a child with a true hyperkinetic behavior syndrome and his normal peer; that is, between a child with a normal and an abnormal central nervous system as the reason for the difference in overt behavior.

Figure 12 shows the results for GSR amplitude, FPV change, and GSR latency. The most striking result is that, in each case, the hyperkinetic child shows very little difference between his autonomic response when he makes a positive or negative response, whereas the normal controls have dramatically

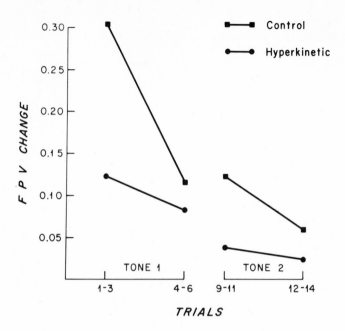

Figure 11.   Changes in finger pulse volume showing lowered responsiveness in hyperkinetics than in matched controls.

higher responses when a stimulus occurs to which they must respond (the "positive" stimulus). If anything, the hyperkinetic tends to show more arousal when the negative stimulus occurs, as though inhibiting his response required more effort than making a response.

To summarize, we may conclude that when appropriately subdivided by clinical characteristics, hyperkinetic children show signs of lower autonomic arousal in response to repetitive stimulation, and less arousal in a "go–no-go" discrimination task.

ALTERING THE CENTRAL NERVOUS SYSTEM IN HYPERKINETIC CHILDREN

The illustrative studies described above, and many others completed in the last decade (Conners, 1974) have provided convincing evidence that hyperkinetic children have lowered arousal levels, central defects in attention and inhibition, delayed habituation of peripheral and central processes; and that certain subgroups exist that are characterized by more or less direct evidence of

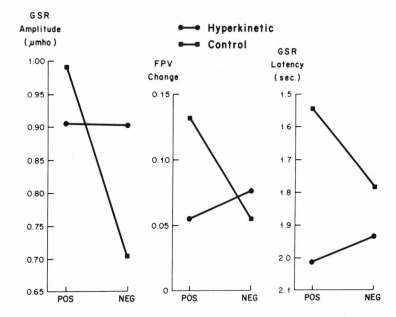

Figure 12.   GSR and FPV responses of hyperkinetic and control children in a "go–no-go" discrimination task. The children must press a key for a high or low tone which is the "positive" stimulus, but must inhibit a response to the "negative" stimulus. Hyperkinetics show much less response change to the two types of stimuli than controls.

neurologic dysfunction (Millichap, 1974) or by distinctive patterns of perform-ance on psychological tests (Connors, 1973).

The use of centrally acting drugs such as the amphetamines and related compounds has been one of the most frequently used treatments as well as tools in the study of the disorder (Connors, 1974). A number of speculations exist about the mechanism of such action, but from a parsimonious point of view it seems reasonable to suppose that stimulant drugs stimulate, and that since behavior is generally "calmed" or integrated, the stimulation must in some sense occur in inhibitory mechanisms of the brain. The fact that the CNS stimulants have a particular affinity for the reticular activating structures of the brain suggests that the increased arousal of these structures (which modu-late cortical tonus and selective attention to external sensory inflow) accounts for the behavioral improvement and apparent cognitive "alerting" effects.

It is now apparent, however, that strong social and ethical forces have made such experimentation much more cautious, and the long-range effects of phar-macotherapy in children have come under increasing scrutiny by the lay and professional public. This no doubt healthy influence has stimulated the search for other methods of altering the central and autonomic nervous system, and the next decade of research will undoubtedly produce novel and interesting methods for changing the hyperkinetic child's nervous system through such techniques as biofeedback, meditation, autogenic training, and other behavioral methods. How might such methods add to our understanding of this group of ill-defined disorders?

One example of new techniques that seems highly appropriate to this problem is the use of biofeedback. In these methods the subject has some portion of his ongoing physiological processes displayed to him, such as his brain waves or his heart rate, and is given information about his changing state with instructions to attempt to alter that state. Viewed from an operant framework, the subject is reinforced for changes that occur in the desired direction. Whatever the internal mechanism by which such "passive volition" operates, it is now well accepted that many subjects can gain significant degrees of voluntary control over physiological processes formerly thought to be completely involuntary or unconscious.

The alpha rhythms of the brain are one such process that can apparently be brought under some degree of voluntary control through the use of feedback training techniques. These electrical rhythms of the brain are large-amplitude, 8–13 cycles per second phasic voltage changes that occur most frequently in the visual cortex of the brain, especially when the eyes are closed and the subject is relaxed. Since these rhythms appear to reflect an "idling" state of the brain, in which large ensembles of neurones are firing in unison or are "synchronized," the reasonable interpretation can be made that these rhythms represent an inhibited state preparatory to information processing. This would have a certain value inasmuch as large ensembles would be orchestrated in the same positive–negative cycle in preparation for stimuli to produce an efficient neuronal response.

It is known that reaction time is faster to stimuli arriving during the negative portion of the alpha cycle (Dustman, 1965), and the period of the cycle (approximately 0.1 seconds) is about the time it takes for a person to switch attention between the two hemispheres in a dichotic listening or vigilance task. It is also known that the cortical evoked response is larger if stimuli arrive during alpha rather than nonalpha periods. (Spilker et al., 1969). If the presence of alpha is related to the efficiency of information processing, and the latter in turn is reflected in the amplitude of cortical evoked responses, then it should be possible to use the visual evoked response (VER) as a measure of cortical efficiency. It seems reasonable to ask whether such efficiency can be increased by teaching the subject to increase his alpha.

A further question is whether the subject can be trained in such a way that he could selectively alter efficiency in one hemisphere of the brain. This would have profound implications for education and behavioral control because of the known specialization of the two hemispheres: the left hemisphere typically subserves verbal, analytic, linear, and discriminative information processing, while the right subserves holistic, geometric, relational, and nonverbal information processing (Gazzaniga, 1967; Bogen, 1969). Nothing is known of hemispheric interrelationships in hyperkinetic children, but there is good reason to assume that in many MBD children either the verbal or nonverbal functions are selectively impaired by maturational lag, brain damage, genetic influences, environmental pollutants, or toxins.

The following experiment on a single child with moderately severe dyslexia is cited as an example of what is likely to become a powerful new research method with MBD children as the alternatives to pharmacotherapy become more available.

In this first experiment (O'Malley & Conners, 1972) the 14-year-old boy had electrodes connected to the left and right occipital regions, and was given a tone signal whenever he produced a burst of alpha that met certain criteria. In addition, the feedback was arranged so that it occurred only when alpha was present in the left hemisphere and either beta or theta rhythms were present in the right hemisphere. That is, the subject had to have a temporary state in which alpha activity was occurring on the left side, while nonalpha was occurring on the right. After each of the 5-minute training sessions, which

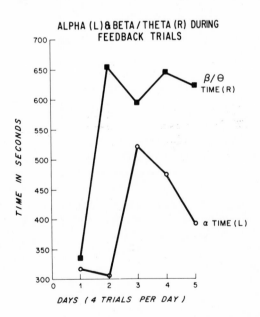

Figure 13. Amount of alpha and nonalpha time on left and right side of subject given feedback for presence of alpha on left when nonalpha occurs on right.

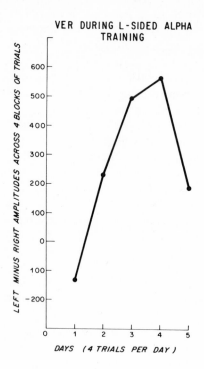

Figure 14. Difference in amplitude between left and right side for visual evoked responses in subject trained to produce higher alpha on left side.

were conducted several times a day over a period of a week, the VER was measured on the two sides of the scalp from the same locations recording the brain rhythms during the feedback experiment.

The changes occurring in alpha, beta, and theta rhythms are shown in Figure 13; Figure 14 shows the parallel changes occurring in the visual evoked response. The changes that occurred are statistically significant for both types of measure, although obviously the findings are limited by the fact of being obtained in this single subject. But the method illustrates the possibility of the kind of research that may make it possible selectively to alter brain states, and hopefully behavioral states, in MBD children.

SUMMARY AND CONCLUSIONS

In this chapter we have argued that the concept of minimal brain dysfunction (MBD) is a useful heuristic concept. The value of the concept is that it has stimulated research into alternative ways of conceptualizing certain childhood disorders as having important bases in the development and function of the central and peripheral nervous system. At the same time that biological domains are explored in the search for causes and mechanisms, the concept of underlying brain dysfunction encourages a shift from purely psychogenic and behavioral methods of treatment towards somatic therapies.

Intrinsic to this shift of emphasis is a pluralistic, polythetic approach to description and measurement of the clinical disorders in which several discrete subtypes or classes are sought, as preliminary to the identification of the different etiologies. A simplistic and reductionistic approach to the biological basis for behavior ignores the interactive relationship between organism and environment, and we have stressed the fact that children with MBD reveal their deficits only under certain conditions of stress or cognitive information processing demand. While somatic therapies such as the use of psychoactive drugs have an important role, newer methods of altering the central and autonomic nervous systems of MBD children hold promise for the coming decade of research and applied investigation.

REFERENCES

Bax, M. The Active and the over-active school child. *Developmental Medicine and Child Neurology,* 1972, **14**, 83–86.

Blau, A. The psychiatric approach to posttraumatic and postencephalitic syndromes. In R. McIntosh (Ed.), *Neurology and Psychiatry in Childhood, Proceedings of the Association.* Baltimore: Williams & Wilkins, 1954, pp. 404–423.

Bogen, J. The other side of the brain. *Bulletin of the Los Angeles Neurological Society,* 1969, **34**, 73–105.

Bond, E.D. & Smith, L.H. Post encephalitic behavior disorders. *American Journal of Psychiatry,* 1935, **92**, 17–33.

Conners, C.K. The effect of dexedrine on rapid discrimination and motor control of hyperkinetic children under mild stress. *Journal of Nervous and Mental Disease,* 1967, **145**, 138–141.

Conners, C.K. Psychological assessment of children with minimal brain dysfunction. *Annals of the New York Academy of Sciences,* 1973, **205**, 283–302.

Conners, C.K. The effect of pemoline and dextroamphetamine on evoked potentials under two conditions of attention. In C.K. Conners (Ed.), *Clinical use of stimulant drugs in children.* Amsterdam: Excerpta Medica, 1974.

David, O. et al. Lead and hyperactivity. *The Lancet,* 1972, Oct., 900–903.

Douglas, Virginia I. Differences between normal and hyperkinetic children. In C.K. Conners (Ed.), *Clinical use of stimulant drugs in children.* Amsterdam: Excerpta Medica, 1974.

Dustman, R. E. & Beck, E. C. Phase of alpha brain waves, reaction time, and visually evoked potentials. *Electroencephalography and Clinical Neurophysiology,* 1965, **18,** 443–450.

Gazzaniga, M. *The bisected brain.* New York: Appleton-Century-Crofts, 1970.

Graham, Frances K. et al. Development three years after perinatal anoxia and other potentially damaging newborn experiences. *Psychology Monographs,* 1962, **76,** 1–53.

Klein, D.F. & Klein, Rachel Gittelman. Diagnosis of minimal brain dysfunction and hyperkinetic syndrome. In C.K. Conners (Ed.), *Clinical use of stimulant drugs in children.* Amsterdam: Excerpta Medica, 1974.

Knobloch, H. & Pasamanick, B. Prospective Studies on the Epidemiology of Reproductive Casualty. *Merrill-Palmer Quarterly of Behavior and Development,* 1966, **12,** 27–43.

Laufer, M.W., Denhoff, E., & Solomons, G. Hyperkinetic Impulse Disorder in Children's Behavior Problems. *Psychosomatic Medicine,* 1957, **19,** 38–49.

Millichap, J.G. & Johnson, F.H. Methylphenidate in Hyperkinetic Behavior; Relation of Response to Degree of Activity and Brain Damage. In C.K. Conners (Ed.), *Clinical use of stimulant drugs in children.* Amsterdam: Excerpta Medica, 1974.

O'Malley, J. & Conners, C.K. The effect of unilateral alpha training on visual evoked response in a dyslexic adolescent. *Psychophysiology,* 1972, **9,** 467–470.

Pope, Lillie. Motor activity in brain injured children. *American Journal of Orthopsychiatry,* 1970, **40** (5), 783–794.

Satterfield, J.H., Atoian, G., Brashears, Gladys C., Burleigh, Allison C., & Dawson, M.E. Electrodermal studies in minimal brain dysfunction children. In C.K. Conners (Ed.), *Clinical use of stimulant drugs in children.* Amsterdam: Excerpta Medica, 1974.

Sauerhoff, M.W. & Michaelson, I.A. Hyperactivity and brain catecholamines in lead-exposed developing rats. *Science,* 1973, **182,** 1022–1024.

Sokal, R.R. Classification: purposes, principles, progress, prospects. *Science,* 1974, **185,** 1115–1123.

Spilker, B., Kamiya, J., Callaway, E., & Yeaker, C.L. Visual evoked responses in subjects trained to control alpha rhythms. *Psychopsysiology,* 1969, **5,** 683–695.

Wender, P.H. & Eisenberg, L. Minimal brain dysfunction in children. In S. Arieti (Ed.), *American handbook of psychiatry* (2nd ed.). New York: Basic Books, 1974, pp. 107–115.

Werry, J. The diagnosis, etiology and treatment of hyperactivity in children. In J. Hellmuth (Ed.), *Learning Disorders,* Vol. 3. Seattle: Special Child Publications, 1968.

PART THREE

Childhood Psychoses

CHAPTER 5

The Experimental Study of Children Vulnerable to Psychopathology*

NORMAN GARMEZY

INTRODUCTION

Aphorisms often provide ingenious summaries of major truths. *"Everyone has a breaking point"* is one such summary of the literature of vulnerability to psychopathology. As such it is not only a part of the naive psychology of the lay public but finds expression in the more sophisticated views of clinical and experimental psychopathologists. The phrase, so applicable to a world at risk, captures a common anxiety of children and adults: a sense of vulnerability when exposed to stressful life events and experiences.

The aphorism bears the hallmark of a *diathesis–stress* formulation of deviance—one so widely accepted that concepts such as *adaptation, coping, defense, resistance,* and *stress* have become the currency of popular exchange. But once having yielded to the attractiveness of the aphorism, its fragility becomes evident. For while many are eligible for breakdown, few are chosen, and those who are seem to capitulate to stresses that run a gamut of intensity ranging from the innocuous to the pernicious.

Vulnerability to psychopathology thus appears to be a threshold phenomenon that implicates a profound individual differences factor. It is the exploration of this variable of individualized vulnerability, whether from a biological,

*This chapter is an abridged but revised version of a longer monograph that appeared in the Schizophrenia Bulletin (1974, #8, 9) (Copyright by Norman Garmezy). Preparation of the chapter was facilitated by several grants: USPHS Contract No. PH43-68-1313, a Research Career Award MH-K6-14, 914, the Schizophrenia Research Program, the Supreme Council 33° A. A. of the Scottish Rite, Northern Masonic Jurisdiction U.S.A., and NIMH Grant MH22836-02 (University of Rochester).

Copyright © 1975 by Norman Garmezy

psychological, or sociological perspective, that constitutes the domain of what is now called *risk research*.

This domain is bounded by two research foci: the study of *predisposition* (i.e., diathesis) and the investigation of *stress* potentiators. The former is indexed by those components of a genetic and/or cultural heritage which either singly or in combination determine the threshold of adaptive responsiveness to specific life experiences. It is these experiences—the vicissitudes of life—which mark the study of stress and its consequences, factors which, in conjunction with predisposition, provide the basis for adaptive or maladaptive personality formation.

The fragility of the "breaking point" aphorism is shared by diathesis–stress theory. Evaluating this formulation in the context of schizophrenia, Rosenthal (1963) has written:

> Presumably, the severity of the disorder depends upon both the degree of inherited predisposition and the degree of stress. . . . Such theories are the ones in which genuine meaning attaches to the commonly repeated statement that heredity and environment interact to' produce schizophrenia. However, as implied, the great majority of them are also exasperatingly loose, since the nature of the predispositions and the stressors, as well as the mechanisms of interaction, are usually only vaguely conceived or formulated. Research strategy here must focus on elucidating these complex issues. (pp. 508–509)

One such strategy is the study of children who may be at heightened risk for psychiatric disorder in later life. Recent developments in the study of such children suggest that we are witnessing the emergence of a research area centered on individual predisposition to psychopathology and the distinguishing modes of coping and adaptation characteristic of those who resist and of those who capitulate to behavior disorders.

This chapter provides a capsule description of some of the ongoing efforts to study the nature of vulnerability in children predisposed to the more severe forms of such disorders, and some of the central research issues involved in investigations of risk potential. The emphasis in the chapter is on predisposition to schizophrenia, but the restriction is an arbitrary one and the lessons to be derived from this seemingly narrow focus have broad applicability to the countless forms of behavioral deviance that plague mankind.

Researchers into vulnerability to severe psychopathology are relative newcomers to a risk scene that has been occupied by other investigators interested in the long-range outcomes of certain disabling tendencies in children. Two examples: (1) delinquency and antisocial behavior have been target concerns of those interested in the pathogenic role played by family and community in heightening the probability of antisocial behavior in adulthood (e.g., Robins, 1966; McCord & McCord, 1959); (2) pediatric researchers and developmental psychogists have evaluated risk potential in followup studies of infants exposed to prenatal and perinatal nutritional deprivations, anoxia, prematurity, birth and pregnancy complications, and the like (e.g., Smith et al., 1972; Harmeling & Jones, 1968; Wiener et al., 1968; Corah, et al., 1965; Dann et al., 1964; Drillien, 1961; Ernhart et al., 1960).

Many of these studies have taken a long- or short-term longitudinal-developmental perspective. By contrast, the study of the precursors to severe psychopathology demonstrates an unyielding emphasis on the retrospections of adults about significant early factors in the lives of already disordered persons.

But the scene is changing and the reasons for such change reflect a confluence of many factors.

The Current Emphasis on Children at Risk

Psychiatry has played favorites. Adults have long been the focus of psychiatric investigation, whereas children have been the victims of a benign neglect. As a result, our knowledge of the structure and the development of mental disorder is built on a rather shaky foundation, a view that was recently described in this way:

Psychiatric clinicians and experimental psychopathologists typically share as their focus of attention the disordered adult patient. Whether one's persuasions are biological or psychological, contemporaneous observations are often used to infer not only the structure of mental disorder but its significant antecedents as well. For the structuralists . . . the focus on the adult informant is appropriate. But for the etiologist such an inferential enterprise poses problems. To suggest that case history information gathered in the present is an accurate reflection of the past—and to do so in the face of many confounding variables—only confuses the scientific effort to untangle causation in psychopathology. (Garmezy & Streitman, 1974, pp. 14–15)

Although clinicians have always monitored adult memories to partial out the effects of a client's motivational and defensive operations, theoretical constructions about the origins of psychopathology nevertheless have been largely based upon those very offerings which, if introduced in the course of a therapeutic hour, would be examined with circumspection.

Such caution seems justified by a variety of observations relating exogenous factors to interpretations of clinical states. Biological researchers, for example, have described the role played by hospital environments, dietary insufficiencies, and inactivity on biochemical variations in patients (Kety, 1959, 1969; Wyatt, Termini, & Davis, 1971). Similarly the psychologically and sociologically minded have pointed to the effects of illness, patienthood, and the hospital milieu on a patient's communications, memory, motivational states, and indicators of personal and social inadequacy. Mednick and McNeil's (1968) cautionary note reflects the problem:

It may be difficult . . . to isolate etiological factors through studies carried out with individuals who have lived through the process of becoming and being schizophrenic. The behavior of these individuals may be markedly altered in response to correlates of the illness, such as educational, economic, and social failure, prehospital, hospital and posthospital drug regimens, bachelorhood, long-term institutionalization, chronic illness, and sheer misery. (p. 681)

These cautions have been joined to other research investigations that are somewhat farther afield. Developmental psychologists have cast into question the veridicality of retrospective accounts as provided by normal mothers of normal offspring. Typically the time span involved in these studies has been far shorter than that demanded of parents of disordered adults asked to reconstruct the early environmental milieu of their offspring. The discouraging findings of the normal developmental studies, therefore, have had a disquieting effect on research psychopathologists. In these normative studies the validity of the parent's reports could be matched against various behavioral records taken during the years that were the focus of inquiry. In most cases the recorders of such data had been professional observers—teachers, physicians, and the like. Perhaps the most carefully drawn of these studies has been provided by Yarrow et al. (1970), who were able to compare mothers' recall of the nursery school behavior of their offspring against cumulative case folder information and behavioral observations that were still available from the nursery school their children had attended some three to thirty years previously. The investigators found not a random bias (that would have been dispiriting enough) but rather systematic ones that cast the validity of the mothers' observations into question. Among these were the following:

1.   An offspring's current adjustment determined the mother's reminiscences and ratings of the past. An adaptive present generated the view of an adaptive past, fusing the life history into an image of trait consistency.

2.   The further removed the offspring was from childhood, the more favorable were the mother's memories of that earlier period.

3.   Reports of an offspring's dominant personality attributes in later years led to the mother's assignment of consistently higher ratings to those qualities during childhood.

4.   Mothers were tied to a Spockian view of the world. As the authors express it: "We found mother's reports conforming to child welfare values current at the time of reporting" reflecting their indoctrination by contemporary "theories of development and behavior."

Such findings scarcely constitute an enthusiastic endorsement for the validity of parents' recall of their children's early years.

Developmental research on the process of socialization further heightened a concern with parental reports of mother-child relationships. By the 1940s and 1950s clinical and experimental studies of the effect of the family on the genesis of schizophrenia in an offspring had become, figuratively, a one-way street of parental blame. The possibility that socialization involved a two-way process in which both parent and child could provide each other with reciprocal negative effects was largely ignored. Only in the more sophisticated research climate of today, has the accumulating research data on socialization revealed the effects children can exercise over parents—effects which cast into question formulations built exclusively around a unidirectional parent-effect model (Lewis & Rosenblum, 1974; Clarke-Stewart, 1973; Bell, 1968; Thomas, Chess, & Birch, 1968).

The view is summed up in Bell's (1968) statement:

. . . parent control behavior, in a sense, is homeostatic relative to child behavior. To predict interaction in particular parent–child pairs it is necessary to know the behavior characteristics of the child, the cultural demands on the parent, and the parent's own individual assimilation of these demands into a set of expectations for the child. (p. 88)

To achieve this aim, researchers must forego retrospective accounts of the past in favor of an ongoing longitudinal-developmental perspective in which the developing child, whether normal, vulnerable, or psychopathological, becomes the center of inquiry.

Other forces have also moved psychopathologists to the study of precursor states and early vulnerabilities to disorder. The first half of the twentieth century has been termed the era of the neuroses, but the last half and particularly the closing quarter of the century belongs to the study of the psychoses. This shift has been brought about by the rising expectations provided by new forms of pharmacological interventions into schizophrenic and affective states and the discovery of likely biochemical underpinnings for the new pharmacalogia. A renascence of biological psychiatry, sparked by advances in genetics, neurophysiology, and biochemistry has given stimulus to the investigation of early predisposing factors in the severe psychiatric disorders.

Interestingly, this emergent biological awareness was matched by a growing social concern in the 1960s with the status of helpless, disadvantaged, and deprived children. Staying the course of social pathology became a goal of the Great Society as the debilitating effects of highly disadvantaged environments on social and cognitive processes came to public awareness.

The growing concern with deprivation and its consequences brought to the fore the deleterious effects induced by other forms of disadvantage—affective deprivation, broken homes, parental loss, genetic anomalies—all factors presumed to be implicated in psychiatric risk.

All of these factors, powerful as they were for arousing interest in vulnerable children, would not have been sufficient to energize risk research were it not for the striking growth of developmental psychology. Here was a revitalized discipline capable of providing new theoretical insights into the process of development as seen in the studies, insights, and conceptualizations of Piaget, joined with the investigative efforts of other developmental psychologists whose theoretical net encompassed learning theories. Developmental psychology held out the hope that it could provide the substantive base for understanding the normal development of psychological processes against which, in time, deviant development could be appraised.

But such processes were not to be studied in vacuo. While the cathexis for the laboratory has remained, the child's world is a naturalistic one and systematic descriptive accounts of children's behavior in naturalistic settings have become a significant part of research into children's adaptations. Interest in the developing child has, in recent years, been fostered by the application of ethological principles to the study of the behavior of children. Professor Tinbergen recently noted (1972) the potential power of ethology when he wrote:

> . . . it is on the one hand surprising how much is being discovered which so far has simply been ignored by the professional psychologists; on the one hand it is clear that this simple, careful observation of normal children is going to be a very demanding task indeed. But it will give wider scope and more purpose to human studies. And, no less important, by gradually building up an ethogram of our species, work such as is represented here will provide the yardstick by which behavior pathology can be measured. The words of Sir Peter Medawar could well have been taken as a motto: " .
> . . it is not informative to study variations of behavior unless we know beforehand the norm from which the variants depart. (Jones, 1972, p. ix)

It is the confluence of these factors—concern for the validity of inquiries into childhood through the medium of adult retrospections, the growing understanding of the nature of psychoses, the replacement of therapeutic despair by hopefulness, concern with deprived children and the cognitive and social consequences of neglect, the emergence of biological psychiatry, developmental psychology, and ethology—that have contributed to the study of risk in childhood to which we now turn our attention.

THE SEARCH FOR CHILDREN AT RISK

Who stands at risk? The answer to that question would be a simple one if our knowledge of the etiology of severe mental disorders were reasonably complete. Since it is not, speculation flourishes and, in Maher's (1966) words, provides a research climate in which "hypothesis struggles with hypothesis in a conflict in which new contenders enter the field but the defeated never retire." We are entrapped within a circle in which we are called on to select vulnerable children on the basis of some reasoned etiological model but such a reasoned state demands stable empirical findings that are in notoriously short supply. And those findings that do exist are often based upon research methods that generate more questions than they answer. Nevertheless, one must take the icy plunge in evaluating the available data on a disorder within the context of specific etiological models. Faith in the viability of a model may be the ultimate criterion by which one selects specific determiners as a basis of choice of children presumed to be more vulnerable (than randomly selected children) to a specific disorder.

We are faced in psychopathology with a field in which many disciplines ranging from sociology to biochemistry can lay legitimate claim that each provides some understanding of the nature of behavioral disorders. If there is one true faith it has not as yet made its appearance, so one is forced to fall back upon critical acumen, scholarly appraisal, and faith, interlarded with a minimum of bias, to select those children in a community presumed to be at risk. Models of etiology that have the soundest empirical base and hopefully a reasonable degree of precision form the basis for our choice, but imprecision in itself does not necessarily imply infertility. As the philosopher Abraham Kaplan (1964) has observed:

> Careful observation and shrewd even if informalized inference have by no means outlived their day. I am not saying that there is any antithesis between richer and rigor, but only that it would be equally wrong to take it for granted that there is necessarily a correspondence between them. If there is a choice to be made, for the empirical scientist there is in fact no choice but to go for the riches. (p. 284)

At this point in our science the choices among models are several and the need for a coexistence of diversity seems in order at least until the predictive power of each model can be resolved. Again Kaplan:

> The dangers are not in working with models, but in working with too few, and those too much alike, and above all, in belittling any effort to work with anything else. (p. 293)

The Range of Etiological Models in Psychopathology

Exposition lends itself to a tabulation of unidimensional models, but multiple causation is the way of life in psychopathology. But as Zubin (1969, 1972), a senior statesman of psychopathology research, has noted, we must consider each unidimensional model in its own right before we contemplate it in interaction with other models. His analogy is that of a statistician performing an analysis of variance, who is aware that none of the main effects are likely to operate independently, but first looks to such effects before moving on to a study of their interaction with other variables.

Adopting this posture Zubin has identified six major models, three of which emphasize internal causation in psychopathology (*genetic, biochemical, neurophysiological*), while for the three others external factors in etiology are stressed (*ecological, developmental,* and *learning and conditioning*). These models are summarized in Table 1.

Table 1.   Unidimensional Models of Psychopathology (Adapted from Zubin 1969, 1972)

A. Causation is internal	
1. Genetic	Mental disorders are produced by the interaction of gene and environment. The basic predisposition is laid down by a genetic component but the range of behavior reactions is related to the nature of the environment (i.e., depriving vs supportive).
2. Internal environment	The sources of mental disorder are found in the organism's internal environment, primarily in its biochemical and metabolic characteristics.
3. Neurophysiological	Mental disorder is related to deviant brain function, particularly in its electrophysiological aspects (e.g., arousal states, defects in orienting behavior, information processing, etc.).
B. Causation is external	
4. Ecological	The source of mental disorder rests in noxious elements in the environment (e.g., poverty, deprivation, discrimination, population density, social disorganization, and social isolation).
5. Developmental	Mental disorders originate in important transitional states in the life cycle; events may inhibit the development of attributes necessary for adaptation at a later stage (e.g., pregnancy, birth defects, severe affect deprivation in infancy may prevent the development of competencies that are prerequisites to later adaptation).
6. Learning and conditioning	Deviant behavior, like normal behavior, is learned. The symptom *is* the disorder and the positing of underlying processes to account for the disorder is unnecessary.

Of the six models that have been described, investigators of risk for severe psychopathology have focused their attention primarily on three models: the genetic, the ecological, the developmental, and have elaborated on a fourth model—a psychogenic one—but expanded beyond the more limited confines of a learning and conditioning paradigm to incorporate a broadened view of psychological etiology.

In the discussion of the models that follow and for the remaining sections of this chapter, the emphasis will be on vulnerability to severe psychotic states in general but with a particular focus on schizophrenia.

The Genetic Model

Of all the models cited, the genetic model provides the most substantial base of empirical data available to those interested in vulnerability to severe psychotic states, and particularly schizophrenia. Criticisms of methodological shortcomings in earlier genetic studies of this disorder have been offset by more recent investigations in which greater precision in the selection of cohorts, a clearer delineation of diagnosis, and creative research designs have been joined to sophisticated statistical analysis to provide a more powerful indication than has hitherto been available of the presence of a genetic factor at least in the case of a more process-like schizophrenia. Among the studies deserving special citation are those of Gottesman and Shields (1972), Kety et al. (1968), Heston (1966), and Fischer (1973).

It is on the basis of such studies that risk status has been accorded to the offspring of schizophrenic parents by most investigators of vulnerability for that specific disorder. The advantages of such a selection procedures are two-fold: (1) the empirical basis for a genetic involvement is sturdier than that of any competing etiological model; (2) the model provides a broader base for selection since the probability of an ultimate outcome of schizophrenia in the offspring of a single schizophrenic parent approximates 12–14%, while that for children born of dual matings shows an incidence rate that falls approximately between 35 and 45%. The critical factors for risk researchers are thus both theoretical and pragmatic. If one is exploring a disorder with a low base rate any procedure that significantly raises that base rate has a logistical utility that can even transcend theoretical advocacy.

The Ecological (Sociogenic) Model

The sociogenic model of risk for schizophrenia has a somewhat anomolous status. The existence of an inverse relationship between incidence and preva- lence rates for schizophrenia and social class position has been sufficiently replicated to establish it as one of the most sturdy of relationships observed in the study of that disorder. Nevertheless the model has been a weak one for defining the criteria involved in selecting children at risk. Children whose parents occupy the lower rungs of the social scale are a heterogeneous lot and to assign a uniform pathogenicity to their environments seems a naive, dis- torted and single-minded interpretation of the correlation between social class and disorder. The controversial nature of efforts to interpret the direction of effect in that correlation has been set forth by Dohrenwend et al. (1970):

Is low social status more a cause or is it more a consequence of psychiatric disorder? On the basis of research to date, it has been impossible to tell: for this relationship can be explained with equal plausibility as evidence of social causation, with the environmental pressures associated with low social status causing psychopathology; or by contrast, it can be explained as evidence of social selection with pre-existing psychiatric disorder leading to low social status. The latter interpretation is compatible with the position that genetic factors are more important than social environmental factors in etiology. (p. 197)

This problem of interpreting the causal chain is compounded by the all-inclusive nature of social class that limits its power as a variable for understanding its role in the genesis of disorder. Since we encounter difficulty in entangling its predispositional contributions, we can inquire into those factors contained within social class status that allow us to accord it status as a stressor. This effort to partial out the dynamics of social class status Block (1971) has termed "psychologizing the social class variable." That social class correlates with many different types of psychological variables (ranging from IQ and other social competence indicators to patterns of child rearing) is well established, but it is equally well established, as Block notes, that "personality variations *within* social classes far exceed the variations *between* social classes." And such relationships, we can anticipate, will become even more attenuated as we move toward an ever greater degree of "cultural homogenization." How then to interpret the relationship of social class to psychopathology, and of greater importance how to use it as a basis for delineating risk potential. A quotation from Block provides the framework for a needed reductionism, while the views of a prominent sociologist allow us a first glimpse of how we might be able to harness the concept of social class to the study of vulnerability in children. First, Block's commentary:

The most that can be expected of the social class variable is that it will serve as an indicator of several sets of influences, measuring none of them well. Accordingly, it is far better to be rid of the notion. For the sake of both predictability and understanding . . . the gross measure of social class should be abandoned and be replaced by separate, psychological measures, each of which would be finely tuned to represent the concepts and influences now so imperfectly conveyed by social class indices. By psychologizing the concept of social class and partitioning it into its proper components, the possibility is developed of achieving strong and invariant relationships between socialization experiences and subsequent personality. (Block, 1971, p. 274)

But what factors are the proper components? The act of simple identification, even in the absence of the fine tuning of such components that would be needed in research, would be a first step toward using the sociogenic model in risk studies.

This first step has been assayed independently by Kohn, a sociologist long interested in mental health issues. With Block, Kohn shares the view that social class lays down for the child very basic orientations to the environment that are derived out of socialization experiences that are class specific (these approximate Block's "uniform social learning contexts") and shape the personalities of children.

In Kohn's analysis such orientations become the components of social class that demand investigation and which may relate to the etiology of schizophrenia:

> Social class indexes and is correlated with so many phenomena that might be relevant to the etiology of schizophrenia. Since it measures status, it implies a great deal about how the individual is treated by others—with respect or perhaps degradingly; since it is measured by occupational rank, it suggests much about the conditions that make up the individual's daily work, how closely supervised he is, whether he works primarily with things, with data, or with people; since it reflects the individual's educational level, it connotes a great deal about his style of thinking, his use or non-use of abstractions, even his perceptions of physical reality and certainly of social reality; furthermore, the individual's class position influences his social values and colors his evaluations of the world about him; it affects the family experiences he is likely to have had as a child and the ways he is likely to raise his own children; and it certainly matters greatly for the type and amount of stress he is likely to encounter in a lifetime. In short, social class pervades so much of life that it is difficult to guess which of its correlates are most relevant for understanding schizophrenia. (Kohn, 1968, p. 164)

The structure of sociogenic theory is, at this point, more scaffolding than brick and mortar. Before we can apply its concepts to studying children at risk it is first necessary to define the components of its principle construct, social class, to derive methods for measuring these components ("fine tuning" in Block's metaphoric language) and then to test the power of these instruments to differentiate risk and control populations. A long and difficult task, but a necessary one if sociogenic hypotheses are to compete with alternative models.

The Psychogenic Model: Families and the Context of Learning

The more traditional learning model as described by Zubin stands in contrast to those biological models that emphasize genetic, biochemical, and neurophysiological mechanisms. Using learning paradigms derived from the laboratory and behavioral analogues provided by animal experiments, advocates of a learning viewpoint emphasize similarities in the mode of acquisition of deviant and normal behaviors. "Symptoms" for the learning theorist, become labeled responses that are acquired in a manner comparable to the acquisition of other types of behavior. For the learning-oriented researcher the model demands a fine-grained analysis of deviant behavior in which are emphasized the specific nature of stimulus events, the operant responses made to such events, the contingent or noncontingent schedules of reinforcements that exist in the environment, and the shaping of adaptive and maladaptive behaviors that follow as a consquences of specific response-reinforcement contingencies.

This type of an analysis of behavior has been frutifully directed toward the already disordered child or adult. But its application to the selection and study of risk samples, to the best of my knowledge, remains a promise more than an actuality. The reason for this neglect does not require extensive search. It arises from our lack of knowledge about the specific types of stimulus events, responses and reinforcement contingencies that conduce to the development of the most severe forms of psychopathology. This is the status of the operant paradigm at present, but the impact of the Skinnerian Revolution certainly provides an expectancy that such an analysis may be forthcoming at some future date. Zubin's (1972) comment is an appropriate one:

The . . . experimental findings from many sources lend weight to the learning model. We can expect, as researchers continue to develop increasingly sophisticated analyses of complex human behavior in learning theory terms, that the learning model of psychopathology will continue to gain in its influence. (p. 290).

However, a model based upon an observational learning or modeling paradigm has not been entirely neglected in the study of vulnerable children. In the research program on risk being conducted at Minnesota, two groups of already disordered children have been used as part of a diversified set of samples of vulnerable children. Based upon Achenbach's (1966) procedure for categorizing clinic children into externalizing (antisocial) and internalizing (anxious, timid, withdrawn, somatizing) types on the basis of their presenting symptoms, a set of studies has been completed detailing the high risk qualities of the "acting-out" group. These children exhibit attentional defects (Marcus, 1972), show marked signs of peer rejection (Rolf, 1972), and are manifestly lacking in self-control (Weintraub, 1973). What is of additional interest about these children is the greater degree of disorganization that characterizes their family backgrounds (Achenbach, 1966; Weintraub, 1973). The presence of comparable forms of parental psychopathology in these families strongly implicates a modeling concept of deviance to explain, in part, the behavior of these children although the absence of genetic studies in such families does leave unresolved the issue of whether a more fundamental predisposition to an antisocial form of deviance may be involved. It is of interest that the disorganization is specific to the externalizing child's family; we have not found this disabling factor in the families of internalizing clinic children.

The high risk potential of externalizers as opposed to internalizing children can be further adduced by a number of follow-up studies of the adult careers of these children (Robins, 1966; Shea, 1972). The results reflect a rather dismal picture of later adaption. In comparison with both their internalizing and normal counterparts, these children as adults show a great frequency of psychiatric disorders, a higher divorce rate, more job instability, and a markedly lessened degree of social competence.

The role of the family brings into focus another form of a psychogenic model that serves to orient some risk investigators to the study of family role patterns and family dynamics (Goldstein et al., 1968; Cromwell & Wynne, 1974). A number of these investigators have drawn their conceptual framework from family studies of adult schizophrenia in which the emphasis has been on the family as a "social system" and in which the key attributes have been disordered communication patterns, disfiguring transactional modes, and unhealthy symbiotic alliances within the family. What is learned in the family, these investigators believe (and here the modeling phenomenon is also apparent), are those faulty modes of thought and affect that inhibit the development of competence skills and hence render the offspring more vulnerable to life's vicissitudes. In the words of Wynne (1969), a major contributor to the literature of family factors in schizophrenia:

> Parental communication deviances, a far more subtle measure than symptomatology, appear to be a far more consistent indicator of schizophrenic symptomatology in an offspring that does symptomatology of the parents. If those parental deviances predate the offspring's symptomatology, they should constitute a good device for identifying the families of preschizophrenics before the diagnosis of schizophrenia has been made.

Investigators with a family orientation to risk factors are less involved in the nature of a diathesis in vulnerable children, if one is presumed to exist, than they are in focusing on familial stressors. These, if not the primary causative agent, are seen as potentiators of severe psychopathology in the child at risk.

The Developmental Model: The Role of Early Neglect

Recent years has seen the growth of a substantial body of research attesting to the role played by such factors as inadequate nutrition, pregnancy and birth complications, birth defects, and poor prenatal and postnatal care on adaptation in early and later childhood (e.g., Birch & Gussow, 1970; Pasamanick & Knobloch, 1961; 1966). The concept of "a continium of reproductive casualty" as suggested by Lilienfeld, Pasamanick, and Rogers (1955) and Pasaminick and Knobloch (1961) has been built upon a set of disorders correlated to complications that range from cerebral palsy to various forms of ego dysfunction. Whether a causal chain exists that would allow for valid predictions of later outcome has been questioned (Sameroff, 1974) particularly if a single variable approach is taken to the problem of predicting for risk.

A more adequate model would appear to be an interactional one that takes account of possible bio-constitutional factors in the infant and the familial environment into which the child has been cast (Thomas, Chess, & Birch, 1968). Such a model is, of course, a combinatorial one (i.e., developmental and psychogenic) and attests to the dangers of oversimplifying one's models even for purposes of exposition.

In a recent research program on high-risk infants, so defined by the psychiatric status of their mothers (high versus low psychiatric status as indexed by number of psychiatric contacts and hospitalizations), Sameroff and Zax (1973a, 1973b) have reported on the interdependence of infant temperament attributes and maternal psychopathology. Major differences in infant temperament were found to exist between a normal control group and the two psychopathology groups, with the latter exhibiting a greater frequency of "difficult temperament" profiles. Such profiles reflect irregularity with regard to feeding and sleep times, nonadaptiveness to new or altered situations, intense negative mood, and avoidant responsiveness to new stimuli. These profiles appear to be related to a set of maternal variables that include maternal anxiety, mother's poor attitudes to pregnancy, the demographic variables of race and social class, and the number of previous children the disordered mother has had. The effect of temperament on subsequent competence is suggested by the relationship reported between difficult infant temperament when measured at four months and depressed IQ test scores at age 2 ½. Sameroff (1974) concludes that this constellation of maternal variables helps to predict difficult temperaments in infants during the first year of life—mothers who are anxious, and view their pregnancy and the child that is to follow with distress constitute risk factors for the yet unborn infant, particularly if the mother is poor and has had a limited education. This is the population to study, urges Sameroff, for those who are interested in developmental factors in risk. It is well to quote the implications Sameroff sees in his *transactional model* in which mother and child contribute to a bidirectional causal view of an infant at risk:

The transactional model that we see begins with a mother stressed emotionally, socially, and economically, who produces a child to whom these stresses are communicated producing in it a difficult temperament . . . The negative characteristics of the child provides little reinforcement for his parents and consequently, unless they are free of other social stresses, they do little for the child in turn. The child's resulting relative incompetence at 30 months does little to elicit more positive treatment from his parents and so it goes, a reciprocal process by which the child and his parents march down the road to a less than positive developmental outcome.

Commenting on the implications for intervention of his proposed model, Sameroff notes that the view that development arises from the transactions that continuously obtain between a child and the environment permits an "optimism that we can find myriad points at which interventions can act to normalize both the child and his environment."

There are two other sources of data that implicate a developmental view of risk for schizophrenia. One is derived from the work of Mednick and Schulsnger and their colleagues (Mednick et al., 1971), who have, for more than a decade, played a central role in the evolution of studies of children at risk for schizophrenia. In a number of published reports based upon their researches of offspring of schizophrenic and normal control women, findings of obstetric complications in risk offsprings have been reported. But, the present status of this variable does not permit a simple summary. On the one hand there are carefully documented reports from the Department of Psychiatry of the University of Lund in Malmo, Sweden of failures to confirm any relationship between severity of maternal mental disturbance and rates of obstetric complications or differences in the physical size of the offspring (McNeil, Persson-Blennow, & Kaij, 1974; McNeil & Kaij, 1974). There is also a more recent report from the Mednick–Schulsinger group (Mizrahi et al., 1974) indicating that the total pregnancy and birth complications (PBCs), as derived from the midwife protocols on 166 of the 207 high-risk subjects and 90 of the 104 low-risk subjects of the original Mednick–Schulsinger group, failed to find differences in total PBCs, in severity of complications, in mean number of PBCs per subject, in a wide ranging set of individual variants of obstetrical complications, or of factors that might be suggestive of such complications (e.g., differential use of anaesthetics, stimulants, etc.). Even the mean birthweights for the high-and low-risk offspring, a report recurrent in the literature, proved not to be significant.

On the other hand, however, there are other recent reports that do seem to implicate developmental deviancies. Rieder and his colleagues at NIMH (Rieder et al., 1975) have issued the first of a series of reports on neurological development or deviant visual-motor impairment suggestive of such dysfunction. In general, the view taken by investigators (Fish & Hagin, 1973; Sobel, 1961; Marcus, 1974, Erlenmeyer-Kimling, 1974) of such deficits have implicated a genetic rather than a developmental model, but these studies are incorporated in this section for two reasons: (1) they bear a strong developmental cast; (2) several appear to suggest the impact of environmental effects on neurological dysfunction.

The variability in the data reported under the developmental model, particularly the recording of defect states at birth and in early infancy, points the way to needed studies of the context and consequence of such early defects. What is required of future investigators of this area is an emphasis on comparative developmental studies of subsets of genetically high- and low-risk groups with and without signs of pregnancy, birth, and perinatal complications. A comparison of longer-range outcomes among such groups might suggest the presence of deficits in behavior that serve as precursors to later more significant forms of maldevelopment.

Table 2. Current Programs of Prospective Research on Children at Risk for Schizophrenia and Related Disorders[a]

Investigator(s)	Locale	Age Range of Children	Criteria for Risk Group Selection	Criteria for Control Group Selection	Central Variables	Effort at Intervention	Central Reference[a]
Anthony, E.J.	St. Louis, Missouri	Preschool School age Adolescence Early adulthood	Schizophrenic mother or father	Parent with physical disorder Parents free of mental or physical disorder	Clinical assessment Home visits Information processing Neurological assessment Piagetian tasks (egocentrism) Play behavior Psychophysiology	Yes	Anthony, 1972
Erlenmeyer-Kimling, L. & Rainer, J.	New York, New York	School age	Schizophrenic mother or father Two schizophrenic parents	One or two parents nonschizophrenic with psychiatric disorder Normal control parents	Attentional tasks Home visits Neurological assessment Physical development Psychiatric assessment Psychological assessment Psychophysiology School evaluations Social behavior	No	Erlenmeyer-Kimling, 1975
Erlenmeyer-Kimling, L. & Rainer, J.	New York, New York	Adolescence Early adulthood	Two schizophrenic parents	Schizophrenic mother; nonschizophrenic psychiatric disordered mother	Attentional measures Birth data Developmental data Electrophysiology Neurological assessment Personality assessment Psychiatric records Psychophysiology School records Visual-motor tasks	No	Erlenmeyer-Kimling, 1968

Fish, B.	New York, New York, and Los Angeles, California	Infancy	Schizophrenic mother		Developmental tasks: arousal autonomic functioning vestibular functioning Neurological assessment Visual-motor tasks Psychological assessment	Yes · Fish & Hagin, 1973 Fish et al., 1966
Garmezy, N. & Devine, V.	Minneapolis, Minnesota	School age	Schizophrenic mother	Depressive mother Acting-out child Withdrawn child Matched and random normal controls hyperactive child	Attentional and vigilance tasks Competence measures Information processing School records Sociometric measures Teacher ratings	No · Garmezy, 1973
Grunebaum, H.V.	Boston, Massachusetts	Infancy Preschool School age	Psychotic mother	Nonpsychotic mother	Attentional and vigilance tasks Cognitive styles Competence measures Mother–child interaction Psychological assessment	Yes · Grunebaum et al., 1974
McNeil, T.F. & Kaij, L.	Malmo, Sweden	Prenatal and infancy	Schizophrenic mother	Matched non psychiatric mother Manic-depressive mother Atypical endogenous psychosis— mother	Birth and obstetrical data Infant temperament Maternal attitudes toward pregnancy Mother–infant interaction Neurological assessment Psychophysiology	No · McNeil & Kaij, 1973

Table 2. (Continued)

Investigator(s)	Locale	Age Range of Children	Criteria for Risk Group Selection	Criteria for Control Group Selection	Central Variables	Effort at Intervention	Central Reference[a]
Marcus, J. and colleagues	Israel	Infancy	Schizophrenic mother or father	Other psychiatric disorders in mother or father Normal control parents	Attentional (visual) tasks Biochemical measures catecholamine metabolism Infant temperament Mother–infant interaction Neurological-behavioral assessment Sleep studies	Yes (projected)	Marcus, 1974
Mednick, S.A. & Schulsinger, F.	Copenhagen, Denmark	Adolescence Early adulthood	Schizophrenic mother	Matched control nonpsychiatric mother	Birth and obstetrical records Clinical assessments: Personality Significant life events Positive aspects of personality functioning Psychophysiology School records Word association tasks	No	Mednick & Schulsinger, 1968
Mednick, S.A. & Schulsinger, F.	Copenhagen, Denmark	Infancy School age	Schizophrenic mother or father	Character disordered mother and father Normal control mother and father	Assessment and vigilance tasks Birth and obstetrical data Home ratings Neurological assessment Pediatric assessment Psychological assessment Psychophysiology	No	Mednick et al., 1971

Author	Location	Age focus	Focus	Sample	Measures		Reference
Mednick, S.A., Schulsinger, F. & Venables, P.	Mauritius, Indian Ocean	Preschool	Specific psycho-physiological patterns of the child	"Normal" psycho-physiological patterns	Operant conditioning Peer relationships Play behavior Psychophysiology Social competence Socialization patterns	Yes	Mednick & Schulsinger, 1973
Miller, D.	San Francisco, California	School age	Psychiatric disorder in parents	Felons (parents) Welfare recipients (parents) Normal controls (parents)	Clinical assessment Court records School functioning Social agency records Social competence	Yes	Miller, 1966
Rodnick, E.H. & Goldstein	Los Angeles, California	Adolescence Early childhood	Differential symptom patterns in disturbed adolescents: a) aggressive, antisocial b) active family conflict c) passive-negative d) withdrawn, socially isolated	Acutely ill schizophrenic patients for contrast purposes	Clinical assessment Coping behavior Family process variables Psychophysiology Social communication patterns Therapeutic change measures	Yes	Goldstein et al., 1968
Rolf, J.E. and colleagues	Burlington, Vermont	Preschool	Schizophrenic parent	Economically deprived parents Unsocialized aggressive children	Epidemiological survey of early behavior disorders Intellectual competence Peer interaction Play behavior Psychological assessment Social competence	Yes	Rolf & Harig, 1974

Table 2. (Continued)

Investigator(s)	Locale	Age Range of Children	Criteria for Risk Group Selection	Criteria for Control Group Selection	Central Variables	Effort at Intervention	Central Reference[a]
Rosenthal, D., Nagler, S., Marcus J., and colleagues	Israel	School age Adolescence	Schizophrenic mother or father (rearing in Kibbutz or nuclear family)	Nonschizophrenic mother or father (rearing in Kibbutz or nuclear family)	Neurological assessment Psychological assessment Psychophysiology Sensory integration tasks Social competence Word association tests	No	Rosenthal, 1971
Sameroff, A.J. & Zax, M. & Babiqian, H.	Rochester, New York	Infancy Preschool	Schizophrenic mother	Depressive mother Personality disordered mother Normal control mother	Attachment behavior Birth and obstetrical records Conditioning studies Developmental schedules Home observations Infant temperament Maternal attitudes Maternal anxiety Mother–child relationships Object conservation Psychophysiology Social development Stranger anxiety	No	Sameroff & Zax, 1973
Schachter, J.	Pittsburgh, Pennsylvania	Infancy	Schizophrenic mother	Other maternal psychiatric disorders Normal control mother	Bayley developmental tests Developmental data Physical growth studies Electrophysiology Home environment studies Maternal care Psychophysiology	No	Schachter, 1974

Weintraub, S. & Neale, J.M.	Stony Brook, New York	School age	Schizophrenic mother or father	Depressive mother or father / Normal control parents	Attentional tasks / Information processing / Psychiatric assessment (parents) / Psychological assessment (parent and child) / Referential communication / School assessments / Social competence / Social interaction tasks	No / Neale & Weintraub, 1972
Wynne, L.C., Cromwell, R.L. and colleagues	Rochester, New York	Preschool / School age	Schizophrenic mother	Other functional psychiatric disorders in mother	Assessments: diagnostic and personality (parent and child) / Conditioning and habituation / Electrophysiology / Family process interaction / Genetic linkage studies / Information processing / Mother (father) child play interaction / Piagetian tasks (role-taking; egocentrism) / Potential genetic markers / Biochemical / Eye tracking / Psychophysiology / Referential communication (mother and child) / School adaptation / School competence / Sensory integration tasks	No / Cromwell & Wynne, 1974

[a] A more complete set of references can be found in Garmezy and Streitman (1974) and Garmezy (1974). The single reference cited in this table typically provides an overview of the project.

SOME ILLUSTRATIVE PROGRAMS OF RESEARCH ON
CHILDREN AT RISK FOR SEVERE PSYCHOPATHOLOGY

In a recent publication (Garmezy, 1974), I have provided extended descriptions accompanied by multiple references of 20 programs of studies of children at risk for schizophrenia and other spectrum disorders. These programs are essentially longitudinal-developmental in design and vary in their theoretical perspective. One can identify those with a marked genetic orientation (e.g., Erlenmeyer-Kimling, pp. 58–63), others with a more psychogenic cast (Rodnick and Goldstein, pp. 78–83), and still others that stress a developmental model (Sameroff and Zax, pp. 86–87). But the range of models used with regard to vulnerability to the most severe psychopathologies has been rather narrow with marked neglect of the three models Zubin has identified as the *ecological,* the *internal environment,* and the *neurophysiological.**

In a forthcoming publication, Erlenmeyer-Kimling (1975) has provided a tabular outline of the most readily identified prospective studies on risk for schizophrenia currently underway. In Table 2, I have taken the liberty of expanding upon her description of these ongoing research programs.

A more extended description of these programs can be found in a recently published two-part monograph on risk research (Garmezy & Streitman, 1974; Garmezy, 1974).

SOME PROBLEMS IN RISK RESEARCH

Selection of Variables

Examination of Table 2 indicates that a wide ranging set of variables are being studied in the projects on vulnerability now underway. The rationale underlying the choice of specific tasks varies, but typically includes the following: First, there are those tasks and procedures that have been shown to differentiate, with consistency, *adult* schizophrenic patients from others, such as meas-

*The neurophysiological model has begun to attract interest as data reflecting psychophysiological and electrophysiological variations in disordered and risk populations have begun to appear. On the basis of their psychophysiological findings with the offspring of schizophrenic mothers, Mednick and Schulsinger (1973) and their colleagues, including Peter Venables, have recently begun a WHO-sponsored research project aimed at primary prevention of severe mental and emotional disorders with high-risk 3-year-old children on the island of Mauritius, off the East Coast of Africa. Risk in this intervention program is defined by deviant patterns of psychophysiological responding in preschoolers comparable to those obtained in Denmark for disturbed offspring of schizophrenic mothers under the broad rubric of the Copenhagen program of risk research.

ures of reaction time, attention, set, and vigilance; information processing tasks including sensory integration measures; psychophysiological measures of arousal, habituation, and recovery rate following onset of a stressful stimulus; electrophysiological studies of average evoked potentials during the course of fluctuations in attention; vestibular functioning; conditioning and generalization; cognitive disturbances as revealed by word association tests; variants in individual cognitive styles; measures of social competence; intellectual competence as adjudged from school records and teacher's ratings; parent–child interaction; deviant patterns of communication manifest in the course of family interaction tasks; referential communication between child and adult; potential genetic markers such as eye tracking dysfunction reported to be present (among others) in adult schizophrenic patients and their relatives (Holzman et al., 1974) and the reduction of monoamine oxidase (MAO) activity in the blood platelets of schizophrenics (Murphy & Wyatt, 1972).

Second, there are those assessment procedures that are designed to measure either fundamental trait dispositions, manifest state disturbances, or developmental lags of a neurological, motoric, or behavioral sort. Included under this rubric would be structured interview procedures to assay current psychiatric status in parents and offspring, tests and interviews to measure personality traits of children, and assessments of neurological and visual-motor functions.

Third, there are variables borrowed by risk researchers from other colleagues whose preliminary investigations suggest they have chanced upon potentially fruitful differentiators. Among these I would include the use of pregnancy, birth, and obstetrical records, and the assessment of significant life events in parents and children.

Finally, there are those variables derived from current research in developmental psychology that reflect lags in social or cognitive development. These would include systematic observation and categorization of mother–child play interaction, the teaching styles of mothers in relation to their children, the use of Piagetian type tasks to measure egocentrism–perspectivism behaviors, evaluations of infant temperament singly and in relation to maternal competence variables, assessments of attachment behavior, stranger anxiety, and socialization patterns, children's performance on attention and memory tasks, language development, assessment procedures to measure physical anomalies and psychophysiological responsivity, and sleep states in the neonate.

This is a wide-ranging set of variables indeed, but the greatest popularity seems to be accorded psychophysiological measures and various tasks designed to measure information processing, attention, and vigilance behavior. The list is a broadly encompassing one, and in the present early state of risk studies such breadth has its virtues. Undoubtedly as more data accumulate, many of these tasks will be dropped in favor of more productive ones.

The Problem of the Continuity of Behavior

The question of behavioral stability is a critical one for risk researchers. Are behaviors stable over time? The answer to that seemingly simple question is a complex one, not easily answered, for it calls into review such factors as the type of continuity involved, the forms of behavior studied, and the ages over which behavioral stability is to be evaluated.

The concept of continuity in childhood embraces three different types involving the twin factors of manifest behavior and its underlying psychological processes (Kagan, 1971). *Complete continuity* is said to be evident when both behavioral stability and comparable processes are involved. It is a relatively latecomer to development being most clearly evidenced in the postpuberty period when the psychological organization of the individual has reached maturity. *Heterotypic continuity* refers to stabilities across two different response modalities that are related to each other by a common underlying process, while, *homotypic continuity* refers to stability in the same response modality. Heterotypic continuity occurs prior to age ten when rapid changes in behavioral systems are taking place. Kagan has provided a correlational example from Bronson's (1967) longitudinal analysis in which boys between the ages of five and seven, who showed marked control and placidity, are shown in adulthood to have narrow interests and conventional modes of thought. The behavior parameters in childhood and adulthood are clearly different, but speculations as to the personality constellation that underlies these seemingly disparate behaviors suggest an oversocialized child who has developed the personality disposition of a timorous, inhibited, and conforming adult.

Homotypic continuity emphasizes comparable behaviors over time, but the superficial similarities may cloak the fact that such behaviors may be in the service of quite different psychological processes, suggesting a developmental lag in expected transformations of behavior that normally occur over time in the cognitive, social, emotional, and motivational domains. It is possible that, particularly in the early years, the failure of a child to show expected behavioral transitions may be an index of vulnerability. Thus, Escalona and Heider (1959) have observed that the persistence of infantile patterns of behavior into childhood is indicative of children who experience subsequent failures in adaptation. If earlier schemata fail to undergo the requisite transformations during transitional stages of development, the child will be unable to cope with the demands and expectancies of a later stage, which itself indicates the "maturational unevenness . . . characteristic of many emotionally disturbed children."

As in the case of intellectual development, the stability of underlying processes that characterize late childhood and adolescence and the instability evident at earlier ages, suggests that there may be an optimal age at which to study risk children. Thus, studies of vulnerable adolescents are likely to allow for the measurement of personality variables with complete continuity; by contrast, the attempt to predict future maladjustment from behaviors exhibited by neonates and preschool children can itself be viewed as a high-risk venture.

TWO PROGRAMS OF RESEARCH INTO VULNERABILITY TO DISORDER IN CHILDREN: THE ROCHESTER AND MINNESOTA PROJECTS

The Rochester Program

The University of Rochester Child and Family Study (URCAFS) is the most extensive study on risk currently underway in the nation. It houses a consortium of 24 collaborating senior investigators, all highly experienced in the core variables they employ, and all focusing jointly on a large group of families at risk, who contribute some 50 hours of participant time to the project. For this account I have leaned heavily on a descriptive report by Rue Cromwell and Lyman Wynne (1974) who serve as the coordinating co-principal investigators of the program (See Wynne, Table 2).

All studies of risk begin with the problem of subject selection. Since the Rochester program is concerned primarily with risk for schizophrenia and related disorders, one of the first issues that had to be resolved was the basis for selecting children who might be particularly vulnerable to such forms of psychopathology. The genetic model suggested consideration of the offspring of parents diagnosed as schizophrenic, but that criterion for inclusion poses a problem that is ubiquitous in the study of vulnerability to severe psychopathology. Cromwell and Wynne write:

> The diagnostic problem with parents in high-risk studies is more difficult because those schizophrenics who become parents are likely to constitute a biased sample, with respect to such factors as sexual experience, marriage, and the raising of children which usually indicates more adequate mental functioning. Thus, diagnostic signs are usually not as distinct as in a random sample of schizophrenics. Especially difficult is the problem when partially or completely intact families are needed for purposes of research design. Simply maintaining stringent criteria is not the answer, since the inevitable outcome is to reduce the number of subjects available for study. On the other hand, relaxing diagnostic criteria does not provide a simple solution either. While sufficient number of cases are then available for investigation, the resemblance of these parents to what we commonly think of as schizophrenics would be even less.

But even relaxing the diagnostic criteria for risk selection does not remove the problem of insufficient numbers of cases. This is particularly true if additional criteria such as social class of the family, race, sex of the disordered parent, family intactness, and age and sex of the targeted offspring are introduced as independent or control variables in the study.

The Strategy of Selection

The Rochester investigative team early considered the use of diagnosed schizophrenic adults and nonschizophrenic (primarily depressive) psychiatric controls as the basis for selection. This traditional view was discarded, however, in favor of including as subjects all those previously admitted to the hospital with a functional psychiatric disorder. An extensive assessment battery of tests and interview procedures is then systematically administered to affirm not merely a diagnosis but to assess other behavioral dimensions that are relevant to the evaluation of risk. This procedure still permits the use of traditional diagnostic categories such as schizophrenia, affective disorders, and the like, but it also allows for evaluation of the concept of a spectrum within these disorders (Rosenthal, 1974) as well as an analysis of dimensions that are known to be predictive of good or poor outcomes in patients (Strauss & Carpenter, 1972, 1974a, 1974b) and which may be related to the degree of risk in the offspring. Examples of such dimensions include process versus reactive status, presence versus absence of thought disorder, paranoid versus nonparanoid symptomatology, acuteness versus chronicity; presence and extent of affective symptoms, variations in social competence, degree of social withdrawal and isolation, etc.

Commenting on this revision in strategy, Cromwell and Wynne write:

> From the point of view of multi-variate analysis and theory development, the flexibility of the strategy . . . is attractive. Not only can single variables, small and large generic groupings of variables, and traditional diagnostic classifications be tested for their efficacy in predicting later breakdown, but, also, newly derived classification systems may be applied.

The Rochester group at the inception of the research program faced the additional problem of deciding on the demographic attributes of the experimental and control groups they would study. The decision was to focus upon male children of white and English-speaking parents who, on the basis of the Hollingshead index, occupied social classes III or IV with extension upward to class II, while specifically excluding the extremes of the social class spectrum (classes I and V). Furthermore, a priority order for the selection of families was established that gave the highest preference to intact families, followed, in turn, by a child living with its mother (father absent), and finally to a child living with father with a mother absent. Specifically excluded from the study, too, were parents who showed evidence of organic brain syndrome, alcoholism or drug addiction, or families in which the mother or targeted child gave evidence of being mentally retarded.

These restrictions were imposed to assure a more homogeneous sample, a decision that spared the investigators one problem while introducing another. Obviously a restricted sample of cases also restricts generalizations that can be drawn from the findings. On the other hand, given the limited numbers of available cases so characteristic of risk studies, any sample that is wide ranging with regard to social class, race, ethnicity, parental ages, and so on generates variance so great as to preclude effective significance tests of the findings. All projects share this common limitation and one can hope that as the number of investigative teams grows, it will be possible to test for data generalizations across investigations and thus, to some extent, overcome the subject limitations of any single project.

Research Design

The longitudinal design used in the Rochester program makes use of a convergence strategy first espoused by Bell (1953) as a compromise between the virtues of a longitudinal design (which permits the study of the stability and predictive power of specific behaviors, traits, and events in the same individuals over time) and those of a cross-sectional design (which can more rapidly suggest the nature of age-related changes in the behavioral parameters under study).

The convergence method (or *short-term longitudinal* or *accelerated longitudinal* design) employs different age groups of subjects who are tested recurrently over relatively short periods of time so that data acquired on them at a given age can bridge into the ages of the older cross-sectional samples in the study.

To the best of my knowledge, the Rochester group has applied this type of design for the first time to the study of psychopathology and its development. The project takes risk and control children (as defined by mothers' psychiatric status) at ages 4, 7, and 10 and hopes to bring them back for repeat testing 3 years later when the groups are then 7, 10 and 13 years of age, respectively. Comparability of performance of the original 7- and 10-year-old children with the younger child groups (ages 4 and 7) 3 years later could suggest the nature of the developmental course in risk samples. In the Rochester study the convergence strategy allows inferences of a probable 9- year span of development, from early childhood to the onset of adolescence, and to do so within a time span of 3–4 years.

From a pragmatic standpoint the decision to apply a convergence strategy to the study of a sample of children at risk stands as a wise one, contingent, of course, on its successful exploitation. That success will depend upon the cooperation of the families involved in the study, their continued presence in the community, and the comparative stability of these families over time.

The Variables Under Study

The assessment and experimental procedures in the Rochester program are extensive, indeed, and require 50 hours of research participation by the collaborating families. Beyond the extended use of case records, and rating scales to record signs and symptoms, there are psychiatric history and assessment schedules that provide a detailed picture of patient, spouse, and family. In addition, more traditional psychological assessment procedures used with both parents range across the spectrum of objective and projective tests and are designed to evaluate intellect, cognitive controls, and the structure of personality. The index child too becomes the object of assessment from both a clinical and interactional viewpoint with part of the procedures utilizing a computerized battery of cognitive tasks that allow for the assessment of the child's psychoeducational abilities.

On the experimental side are to be found procedures that reflect Piagetian theory with its attendant stage concepts, including tests of egocentrism–perspectivism and social role-taking skills. Referential communication games specifically oriented around stimuli that are objective and impersonal are varied with others that require the interpretation of affective states and the use of word association skills that require mother and child to alternate as senders and listeners of word clues in a manner that parallels the seminal work of Cohen and his associates (Rosenberg & Cohen, 1966; Cohen & Camhi, 1967; Cohen, Nachmani, & Rosenberg, 1974).

Family interaction is studied in detail employing a number of procedures with which the names of Wynne and Singer are prominently identified. In addition, Alfred and Clara Baldwin utilize a mother–child play interaction situation they have developed which employs a computerized interaction coding system to analyze many aspects of the play relationship: activity level, warmth, hostility, direction of effects in parent–child exchanges, evidence of support, control, coerciveness, autonomy, dependence, compliance, affect expressiveness, and other types of interactional components that are characteristic of parent and child. This provides the research group with a picture of the stability, the competence, and the cognitive strategies employed by the mother in a naturalistic free-play situation.

Contrasting with the greater freedom of the interactional procedures are the more precise measures derived from the studies of a psychophysiological investigative team that has as its aim the assessment of autonomic variables in parent and child. Studies of habituation, using GSR and heart rate response to meaningless and noxious stimuli, measures of generalization of conditioned autonomic responses, and of average evoked responses to relevant and irrelevant stimuli, are part of this team's efforts to derive a picture of the specific patterns of psychophysiological and electrophysiological responsiveness in parent and child.

In another domain, studies of the child's ability to process information in tasks demanding sensory integration and perceptual scanning are under the direction of a research pair that also conducts extensive studies of the index child's adaptation to school and to peers. The important goal here is to derive measures of social and economic competence in the child's primary work setting, the classroom. The active collaboration of a cooperative county-wide school system has made available to the investigative team critical measures of the index child's adaptation to a world that extends beyond home and family.

The final step is a clinical session with a distinguished clinical psychiatrist who is "blind" to the psychiatric status of the family. In this two-hour session an interview with spouse and former patient focuses on the parents, the patterns of stability and instability characteristic of the family, diagnostic indicators, and, of very great importance, is designed to provide parents with an opportunity to reflect on their research experiences, to clarify and to have answered their many questions, and to provide support and reassurance to them. Such supports are the building blocks derived out of the responsibility, concern, and involvement of the investigators that permits families to contact the staff for assistance and hopefully will facilitate their return to the project 3 years hence.

One-third of the 180 families that will constitute the total sample to be studied have either now been fully seen or are in the process of completing their initial participation in the project. To those familiar with risk studies, publication inevitably is slowed, because of the slow accretion of data. The next several years should begin to witness publication by the various investigative units of the results of their studies, with reports of the efficacy of the convergence design for the study of children at risk.

Project Competence: The Minnesota Studies of Vulnerable Children

Modesty characterizes the Minnesota project when viewed against the breadth and diversity of URCAFS. Whereas most risk research programs are typically longitudinal in design, the Minnesota studies tend to be cross-sectional, employing different children of different ages for the various studies in progress. In additiition, a broader basis is used for selecting a range of risk groups for study. There are four such groups: two groups consist of children who have a greater and a lesser potential for later psychopathology on the basis of the magnitude of the mother's psychiatric disorder; the mothers of the higher potential group have received a diagnosis of schizophrenia; the mothers of the lower potential group have received nonpsychotic diagnoses, of which the major grouping is that of depressive neurosis while in a smaller number of cases some nonschizoid personality disorders are included.

Two other groups of risk children are selected from the case files of community child guidance clinics on the basis of the type of behavior problem that brought them to diagnosis and treatment. Here, too, prognostic potential has been a factor in selection. On the basis of an extensive literature review (see Achenbach, 1966; Garmezy & Streitman, 1974, pp. 45–49), these clinic children are separated into internalizing (good prognosis) and externalizing (poor prognosis) types (Achenbach, 1966). The former typically present complaints of fearfulness, phobias, somatic complaints, shyness, and withdrawal, whereas the latter come to the clinic's attention because of their antisocial or hostile behavior. These children are typically disobedient and destructive, fight with other children, lie, steal, swear, run away, and engage in other depredations that often are correlated with a poor outlook for the future. Figure 1 provides a summary of the origins of the target groups and their prognoses as derived largely from a literature review. A cautionary note, however, is in order. The literature of outcomes for disturbed children indicates that predictions must be tempered with an awareness of the marked variability within such groups that have been noted in followup studies. There are indications that the outcomes for groups of externalizing and internalizing children differ, but intragroup variations are marked and the prediction error is high.

More recently, a fifth targeted group of hyperactive clinic children (who are not on drugs to control their hyperactivity) has been added to provide a contrast with the two clinic groups traditionally used in the project studies.

Selection basis

		Children of disordered mothers	Disordered (clinic) children
Group prognosis	Poor to moderate	Group 1 Psychiatric status of mother: Schizophrenia	Group 3 Clinic status of child: Externalizers (acting–out behavior)
	Moderate to good	Group 2 Psychiatric status of mother: (Primarily) nonpsychotic depressive states	Group 4 Clinic status of child: Internalizers (fearful, anxious, withdrawn behavior)

Figure 1. Four target groups of children at risk in the Minnesota studies.

These target groups of children are initially located in their respective school classrooms from which two control children are then selected. These are children seen as adaptive by school personnel. One child is matched to the target child on the basis of age, sex, grade, social class, family intactness, and achievement and intellectual level whenever possible; a second child, matched only for sex and grade, serves as a random control. On this basis, there are available for statistical study triads of children (target, matched control, and random control) who are distributed over far-flung sectors of a large city.

In our studies we have focused on the years of middle childhood by selecting children from grades 4–6 with occasional incursions into the junior high schools to evaluate seventh and eighth graders. Typically, the numbers of children studied have been quite substantial. In one study (Rolf, 1972), 113 classrooms and 362 children participated; in another (Marcus, 1972), the count was 80 classrooms and 240 children.

The Research Design

The basic approach of the Minnesota project to the study of vulnerable children is contained in a four-stage strategy of research in which a twin emphasis is given to (1) the description and measurement of competence qualities in children, and (2) the search for response parameters that can differentiate adaptive and maladaptive children within risk groups as well as between risk and nonrisk samples. The strategy takes the following form.

Stage 1: Age-Related Indices of Competence

Defining and measuring competence is one of the first priorities in studying the presence in children of precurors to an adult disorder characterized typically by low levels of competence in the premorbid state, delayed onset of the disorder, and a relatively low base rate of its occurrence. Since some forms of schizophrenia show clear prodromal signs in childhood and adolescence, the use of intermediate outcomes (i.e., adaptive versus maladaptive patterns of behavior in childhood) from which to infer successful or unsuccessful adaptation later in life would appear to be a strategically viable procedure.

The problem lies in deciding which attributes best define competence at different ages. Our first approximation to this problem has been to screen children in terms of the characteristics possessed by stress-resistant ("invulnerable") children on the assumption that they are the best exemplars of competence in the presence of risk factors.

Stage 2: The Selection of Response Parameters

The second stage of research involves the selection of response parameters that best differentiate between and within the adaptive and maladaptive members of risk and control groups. Such Stage 2 studies presumably would include those variables that have had significant predictive power in differentiating disordered from nondisordered adults. Thus, in the case of risk for schizophrenia, one can anticipate the inclusion of psychophysiological and electrophysiological variables, measures of information processing, set and attention, evaluations of cognitive efficiency, etc. Other variables may be suggested by normative behavioral studies of children that provide a basis for revealing developmental lags that may be precursors to more severe forms of adaptational failures at older ages.

To test the effectiveness of a Stage 2 study, a Stage 1 competence measure is incorporated in the design to evaluate whether variations on the response parameter correlate with children's levels of achieved competence.

Stage 3:   The Short-Term Prospective Study

The third stage in risk research involves the use of several of these response parameters in short-term prospective studies of children's adaptation. The convergence strategy used in the Rochester program is one such example of a relatively short-term study aimed at an approximation of the developmental characteristics of children at risk and their normal control counterparts.

Stage 4:   Intervention

The ultimate goal of risk research is effective primary prevention. Were the goal to be secondary prevention—that is intervention efforts to ameliorate the condition of an already disordered child—one would expect a traditional therapeutic format to be used. But this is not the type of intervention to which I allude in this stage strategy of research. Rather, the emphasis for primary prevention would be the introduction of experimental and clinical procedures designed to modify a Stage 2 response parameter and then to examine its effects on a Stage 1 competence factor.

Some hypothetical examples may be of particular interest to clinicians involved in working with vulnerable children. Suppose one were to determine that the effective deployment of attention is a significant Stage 2 variable, meaning that vulnerable children show deficits in performance, controls do not; and the presence of deficits appears to be correlated with other indices of maladaptation. An intervention strategy under these circumstances might be aimed at training risk children in more effective attention-focusing strategies. The test of the effectiveness of such training (which would not be a short-term, minimal training experience, but, rather, would require an intensive training commitment), if successful, could then be evaluated against this significant criterion: Does training lead to positive shifts in competence in the trained child in comparison with control children and other risk children not exposed to the intervention effort?

A Digression: Intervention in the Context of a Stage Strategy of Research

Concrete examples of intervention efforts such as the hypothetical one described above are in scarce supply, not only in the study of risk but in the broader domain of clinical activity. However, an example that is available may make this presentation of an abstract research strategy more concrete and more challenging for clinician and researcher alike. Hopefully this will justify this digression.

Earlier in this chapter in referring to methods for selecting variables for use in risk studies, reference was made to the potential significance of developmental lags as possible precursors to later maladjustment. My Rochester colleague, Michael Chandler, and his associates (Chandler, 1971, 1973; Chandler, Greenspan, & Barenboim, 1974) have been engaged in studying Piaget's concepts of egocentrism–perspectivism and role-taking skills as indicators of adaptation and maturity. Social role-taking behavior (i.e., being able to assay the role of another) may well be one dispositional attribute of a maturing individual. All children initially are egocentric in their preoccupations, and as such are unable to differentiate themselves from others. As children grow, this earlier exclusive concern with their own very personalized views of the world is replaced by the ability to recognize and to appreciate the viewpoints of others. Thus, a lag in the acquisition of such role-taking skills, denotes immaturity—a relationship that Chandler has confirmed by testing children who have been institutionalized for emotionally disturbed, antisocial behavior. The correlation between this developmental lag and maladaptation suggests that role-taking may be a significant behavior to study in risk and nonrisk children. Its developmental emergence in normal children and the delayed time table for its appearance in emotionally disturbed children of lesser competence establishes that role-taking skills (or perspectivism) meet the criteria required of a Stage 2 dispositional parameter.

In a series of three studies, Chandler and his group set out to modify this deficit in disordered children using a rather ingenious training strategy as their primary intervention technique. To reduce the deficiency in the targeted sociocognitive skill, an intensive 10-week experimental training program was initiated in which one group of delinquent children were trained to create and to film dramatic video tapes of brief skits that required a rotation among group members of the roles to be played as well as for the technical task of filming the drama. A control group of children made a video taped documentary of their city over the same 10-week span but were denied the opportunity to be role-participants within the film itself. A third group of children served as a control group that had none of these creative experiences available to them.

Results of this unique intervention effort produced enhanced competence in role-taking skills of children who had participated in the self-created dramas, an effect not found in the other two groups. Furthermore, significant behavioral improvements within the institution and in post-institution social adjustment characterized the experimental group in comparison with the two control groups.

In a subsequent study (Chandler et al., 1974), training through the medium of communication games with similar groups of institutionalized children appeared to enhance referential communication and this, in turn, was associated with improvements in social adjustment as judged by staff members of the residential institution that housed the children.

Central Variables of the Minnesota Project

In keeping with the four-stage strategy for risk studies, the Minnesota investigators have focused their efforts on evaluating (1) the competence qualities (Stage 1) and (2) the attentional processes (Stage 2) of vulnerable children.

Initially, we sought descriptive indices of competence and turned our attention to the behavioral correlates observed in children of poverty who showed marked signs of achievement within their school settings. Some have argued that such correlates inevitably reflect middle class values. Perhaps they do, but our counter to that assertion is that children who, in the face of economic adversity, continue to show highly adaptive behaviors are the best providers of information about the sustaining of competence under stress. Furthermore, the correlates to their achievements extend beyond the school into neighborhood and family, thus providing a broader picture of adaptation in the presence of adversity. Should we discard these children because they share the qualities of others who live under more advantageous economic circumstances? To do so would befriend ideology at the expense of knowledge and understanding.

Our view is consistent with one espoused by Connolly and Bruner (1974) in their recent report of a conference on the growth of competence in infancy and childhood:

There probably is no single "position" that would serve to deal with the variety of the impact made by poverty and powerlessness on the life of growing children. But several things were clear in discussion and should be marked in our postscript. One is that it is plainly inaccurate and misleading as well as unprofitable to think of poverty and its impact as a form of impoverishment or deprivation, a kind of "avitaminosis" of culture. Rather, human beings in tough surroundings having to make do with a high chance of failure, adapt ways of covering themselves, trimming aspirations to a point where they protect against disappointment and further setback. . . . It was plain in our discussions, as in much informed contemporary public debate, that programmes of action in behalf of the young caught in the poverty cycle could not be simply "cognitive" or "skill orientated," much of the problem has to do with how one instills a feeling of being in control of one's own destiny, rather than feeling a victim. (p. 311)

Part of that search for control over a world these children of poverty did not create would, in part, be derived out of healthy and more positive expectancies that arise out of self-achievements. It was this view that led Keith Nuechterlein, of our research group, to a search through a largely unpublished literature for data on *The Competent Disadvantaged Child* (K. Nuechterlein, 1970; Garmezy & Nuechterlein, 1972); out of it emerged our first approximation of the criteria of competence that could be used in Stage 1 studies. In abridged form these were:

1. Effectiveness in work, play and love; satisfactory educational and occupational progress; social adaptation as indexed by peer regard and friendships.

2. Healthy expectancies that "good outcomes" will follow when effort and initiative has been imposed on a problem.

3. Self-esteem, and feelings of personal worthiness; a sense of "fate control"—the belief that one can control events in the environment rather than being a passive victim.

4. Self-discipline as revealed by an ability to delay gratification and to be future-oriented.

5. Control and regulation of impulsive behavior; the ability to adopt predominantly a reflective-cognitive orientation to problem situations rather than an impulsive-affective style.

6. The ability to think abstractly and flexibly in approaching new situations and to attempt alternative solutions to a problem.

Studies of Competence

Competence criteria 4 and 5 have been examined by Weintraub (1973), who measured delay of gratification, reflection-impulsivity, and foresight and planning in comparing clinic children with externalizing and internalizing symptoms as measured by the Achenbach Symptom Check List (1966), with a normal control group of children. All three groups were equally divided into lower and middle class social groups as determined by the occupation and education level of the head of each household (Hollingshead, 1957).

Reflection-impulsivity was measured by a more dramatically presented variant of the Matching Familiar Figures (MFF) test, devised by Kagan et al. (1964). The original MFF pictures were photographed and converted to slides that were then projected in an apparatus that made use of buttons and lights as the subject engaged in the task of scanning and matching to a standard stimulus picture.

A measure of foresight and planning was provided by a more traditional assessment instrument, the Porteus Maze Test.

An apparatus used to measure delay of gratification warrants description since it proved to be so intriguing for children. With toys as the choice objects in the delay task a rough equal-appearing interval scale of toy preference was created for use in the experiment. Participating children also indicated their own personal heirarchy of preference by rank ordering each of the 11 toys that were finally used in the study.

The delay of gratification apparatus allowed for a presentation of successive trials of two-choice alternatives that were available to the child (the lesser preferred toy could be taken that same day, the more preferred one could be secured in the principal's office 2 weeks later). Test trials consisted of the presentation of color photographs of the toys in the windows of an apparatus that opened and closed as the child moved a lever along a channel set below the windows. Choice decisions were placed on a card following each trial and at the completion of all trials, a bingo board with disks specified the winning trial, the toy selected and the delay period chosen.

By pairing the toys in terms of their placement within each child's preference hierarchy, a conflict in decision-making could be heightened or reduced. Weintraub reasoned that minimal separation in preference (two very high or two very low preference choices) would produce nondelay in most children irrespective of their group membership, just as maximum separation (a very high preference choice paired with a very low one) would be expected to induce delay behavior in the majority of the subjects.

By contrast, intermediate levels of separations would, Weintraub hypothesized, reveal the tendency to more immediate gratifications presumed to be more characteristic of disordered children.

The results confirmed these expectations. On all three measures, the externalizing children exhibited the least control of all, the internalizing clinic children occupied an intermediate position, but one significantly separated from their externalizing counterparts, while the normal children showed the greatest ability to delay gratification even on the more trying conflict trials.

A particularly interesting finding was the absence of reliable differences between the middle class and lower class normal control children. This finding provided us with empirical support for a view now strongly held by the research group, namely, that *competence transcends social class status.*

A subsequent study by Rolf (1972) examined the social competence of the four target groups and two control groups typically studied on the project, with the social competence measure that of peer acceptance. Rolf used Bower's (1969) technique of casting an imaginery school play with the assignment of positive and negative roles used to infer sociometric standing. With the collaboration of 113 teachers in the same number of classrooms in 37 different elementary schools, data were collected on almost 3000 children who made approximately 60,000 judgments of their peers.

A child's sociometric status is powerfully related to adaptation—a finding that has been consistently reported in the literature and more recently strikingly reaffirmed in a 11–13-year followup of children initially seen as first and third graders in the Rochester Primary Mental Health Project (Cowen et al., 1973). This project is devoted to the early identification of "vulnerable" children and the effects of their subsequent inclusion in a preventively oriented school mental health program. A recent report indicates that not only did these "vulnerable" children subsequently show a disproportionately higher frequency of later appearances in a community-wide psychiatric register, but that the peer judgments, as indexed by the Class Play procedure years previously (third grade), were the "most sensitive" indicator of later maladaptation.

At Minnesota, we *never underestimate the predictive power of a peer* in the study of vulnerability; Rolf's findings reaffirmed that judgment. His data comparing peer judgments made of members of the triads composed of one of four target children (offspring of a schizophrenic mother, depressive mother, clinic externalizers, clinic internalizers) and their respective matched and random controls reveals an order of increasing competence (low to high) of the groups as follows: Externalizers (consistently the least socially competent children); children of schizophrenic mothers; internalizers; children of depressive mothers; and control children, (both matched and random) who were consistently the highest in peer acceptance.

In a subsequent analysis of cumulative school records, Rolf and Garmezy (1974) have reported (as an additional measure of work competence) that all target groups had, at some time in grade school, achieved significantly lower grades than did the controls. Their data also suggest some validation of our initial assumption that risk status varies within the four target groups with children of schizophrenic mothers more closely resembling externalizing children, whereas the offspring of nonpsychotic, depressive mothers, despite manifestations of some behavioral disturbances and school difficulties, most closely resemble the control children.

Stage 2:   The Study of Dispositional Parameters in Vulnerable Children

A Stage 2 study in the research strategy outlined earlier in the chapter requires selection of a response parameter that has a highly stable, dispositional quality which presumably is related to the development of competence in children. The parameter we have studied most intensively relates to attentional processes in vulnerable children as measured by laboratory tasks and in the naturalistic setting of the classroom.

One approach of our group is exemplified by a study conducted by Marcus (1972), who essentially replicated the classic study of reaction time carried out by Rodnick and Shakow (1940) at the Worcester State Hospital more than three and a half decades ago. In this investigation, Marcus tested 240 children using the four types of target children and the two groups of controls characteristic of the Minnesota project. He drew half of his children from the elementary schools (grades 5 and 6) and half from junior high schools (grades 7 and 8), dividing the groups equally by sex and grade status.

The task was a simple auditory reaction time procedure conducted under a regular and irregular procedure using preparatory intervals (PI) of 1, 2, 4, 7, and 15 seconds. To evaluate the modifiability of any performance deficits that might appear in the different groups, Marcus added two additional conditions: one procedure provided the child with a more adequate set of expectancies by informing him/her during the irregular procedure about the length of the PI that would be forthcoming on the following trial. This provided a form of "cognitive facilitation" for the child. Then, to test the consequences of heightening the child's motivation a risk-taking, high-incentive procedure having the aspect of a gambling game (with the payoff for speed a desired toy) was used to supplement the information given the child about the length of the preparatory interval for the next trial. This condition allowed for both cognitive and motivational facilitation. Marcus's results are strikingly conveyed in Table 3.

This table reveals that the various groups of target children, except for the children of schizophrenic mothers, come up to normal performance but under differing test conditions. Thus, for all conditions, internalizers (as in many of our studies) can not be differentiated from their respective controls. By contrast, the comparative attentional deficit that Marcus had posited for children born to schizophrenic mothers remains, despite efforts to provide cognitive and motivational aids. The externalizing children rise to the occasion when presented with a dramatic appurtenance and the incentive of a gambling game but are otherwise unreceptive to assistance in the form of information about the delay period to be anticipated in a test trial. As for the children of depressive mothers, the imposition of minimal additional structure on the reaction time task helps them to achieve parity with their controls. Thus, degree of risk status seems to accompany adequacy of performance in a task that measures attention and information processing mechanisms. The greater difficulties evidenced by children of schizophrenic mothers under all procedures, despite their manifest cooperativeness (which Marcus rated in several ways) may point to a subtle defect in some aspect of the information processing system in these children. Only further research can clarify this important hypothesis.

An ongoing study of vigilance using signal detection theory (K. Nuechterlein) in which target and control groups are to be tested under conditions of incentive motivation and training in cue utilization, hopefully, will help to demonstrate the reliability of Marcus' findings and clarify alternative interpretations of the deficit performance of the higher risk groups.

Table 3. A Schematic Diagram of Attentional Deficits and Nondeficits in Reaction Time Performance Exhibited by Vulnerable Children Relative to Their Combined Matched and Random Controls Under Four Experimental Procedures (from Marcus, 1972)

Deficit Performance X = Deficit (Target > Controls)					Nondeficit Performance 0 = No Deficit (Target = Controls)			
Target Groups[a]					Target Groups			
Higher Risk		Lower Risk			Higher Risk		Lower Risk	
1	3	2	4	Experimental Procedures	1	3	2	4
X	X	X		Regular				0
X	X	X		Irregular				0
X	X			Cognitive facilitation			0	0
X				Motivational facilitation		0	0	0

[a] Higher risk groups: 1 = Children of schizophrenic mothers
                         3 = Externalizers
   Lower risk groups: 2 = Children of depressive mothers
                         4 = Internalizers

A CLOSING COMMENT

The study of vulnerable children has an urgency characteristic of all research that touches on great public health problems. Certainly childhood disorders and children's potential for later disorder is one such problem. The 1970 census reveals a nation of 50,000,000 minors who constitute 26% of our population, one-half of whom are under 10 years of age. Combine these statistics with reports from the National Health Education Committee that 10% of all school age children have emotional problems that require psychological intervention; that the number of boys between the ages of 10 and 14 in mental hospitals increased sixfold between 1950 and 1970, during which time our general population only doubled; that children now comprise 34% of the total case load of outpatient psychiatric facilites—and the depth and the magnitude of the problem of youth amidst disorder becomes evident.

Camus once wrote:

Perhaps we cannot prevent the world from being a world in which children are tortured. But we can reduced the number of tortured children.

Torture comes in many forms—and severe mental disorder is one of the most debilitating, frightening, and malignant forms of all.

There is something particularly poignant about the suffering of children and adults who have been permanently incapacitated by mental disorder. And so

I choose to close this chapter on a personal note by quoting at length from a book, *Wasted*, written by a dear friend of mine, Bill Chapin, in which he chronicles the development of schizophrenia in his son. Toward the end of his book, searching for an explanation for his son's illness—an explanation that eludes us all—Chapin (1972) asks:

What went wrong? We search endlessly for answers, and endlessly we are turned back.

It seems to me it should be obvious that I do not know what went wrong, and neither do the doctors. The doctors can help, they can alleviate, they can exercise certain controls, they can look carefully and deeply into a million minds; but they cannot say, for sure, what went wrong. The good ones cannot, that is . . .

Meanwhile, I can guess, I can suggest.

I think that heredity may have more to do with it than environment. It is easier to blame environment, and that can lead one astray. A persuasive argument can be made that Mark, through his heredity on my side of the family, was born with a predisposition toward mental illness. Several decades ago mental illness was something *other* people had; and it was kept hidden, behind shuttered windows. What the people in my family had was "eccentricity," which was not only condoned, it was often admired. I think, rightfully so; everyone shouldn't be like everyone else.

But was it always just eccentricity? When I was a child I heard one of my mother's brothers referred to as "brilliant," "unpredictable," and "a smart aleck." Indeed he was brilliant: when he was eight years old he wrote a full-length novel about a cat. His mind was an encyclopedia. As a child I was often compared with him, and I deeply resented it. I did not want to have his smart-aleck traits. I now believe that this man, my uncle, who left society to embrace a series of esoteric religions, was eventually a schizophrenic. A parallel can be drawn between his intellectual precocity and Mark's.

Another uncle, a professor at the University of Vermont and one of the nicest of men, committed suicide at a relatively early age.

My father's father spent years in a mental institution, and died there. He had to be "put away" as the expression used to go. Within the family it was never discussed. I can't even remember how I first heard about it, or when.

When my sister had her emotional breakdown at the end of World War II, she went to Montreal to receive expensive treatment, and she recovered. . . .

As I write this, it sounds too much like exhibitionism. Here we are, the crazy Chapins with all their frailties! Exposing all the things that are supposed to be hidden lest someone be embarrassed! But damn it, keeping them hidden hasn't accomplished much. The world's a nutty place. Maybe if we (and by "we" I mean a great many people) stop trying to keep our frailties hidden and stop being ashamed of things we cannot change, the scientists and the doctors *will* discover the causes of schizophrenia, and a cure for it.

And what a blessing that would be; not only for the Mark Chapins of the world, but for everyone. (pp. 211–214)

Chapin's wish is shared by those who study children who are at risk for psychopathology. Our current gropings reflect primitive first steps toward understanding the nature of vulnerability in these children. Hopefully, in time, a more sophisticated awareness of the qualities of the risk child will enable us to reduce the stresses to which he or she may be subjected, or better yet, it may provide us with the methods that will help these children develop more effective ways of coping with adversity.

REFERENCES

Achenbach, T.M. The classification of children's psychiatric symptoms: a factor analytic study. *Psychological Monographs,* 1966, **80** (7); Whole No. 615.

Anthony, E. J. A clinical and experimental study of high-risk children and their schizophrenic parents. In A. R. Kaplan (Ed.), *Genetic factors in schizophrenia.* Springfield, Illinois: Charles C Thomas, 1972, pp. 380–406.

Bell, R. Q. Convergence: An accelerated longitudinal approach. *Child Development,* 1953, **24,** 142–145.

Bell, R. Q. A reinterpretation of the direction of effects in studies of socialization. *Psychological Review,* 1968, **75,** 81–95.

Birch, H. G. & Gussow, J. D. *Disadvantaged children: Health, nutrition, and school failure.* New York: Harcourt, Brace and World, 1970.

Block, J. *Lives through time.* Berkeley, California: Bancroft Books, 1971.

Bower, E. M. *Early identification of emotionally handicapped children in school.* Springfield, Illinois: Charles C Thomas, 1969.

Bronson, C. W. Adult derivatives of emotional expressiveness and reactivity control: Developmental continuities from childhood and adulthood. *Child Development,* 1967, **38,** 801–818.

Chandler, M. J. Egocentrism and childhood psychopathology: The development and application of measurement techniques. Paper presented at the biennial meeting of the Society for Research in Child Development. Minneapolis, Minnesota, March, 1971.

Chandler, M. J. Egocentrism and antisocial behavior: The assessment and training of social perspective-taking skills. *Developmental Psychology,* 1973, **9,** 326–332.

Chandler, M. J., Greenspan, S., & Barenboim, C. Assessment and training of role-taking and referential communication skills in institutionalized emotionally disturbed children. *Developmental Psychology,* 1974, **10,** 546–553.

Chapin, W. *Wasted.* New York: McGraw Hill, 1972.

Clarke-Stewart, K. A. Interactions between mothers and their young children: Characteristics and consequences. *Monographs of the Society for Research in Child Development,* 1973, Serial #153, 38 (6–7).

Cohen, B. D. & Camhi, J. Schizophrenic performance in a word communication task. *Journal of Abnormal Psychology,* 1967, **72,** 240–246.

Cohen, B. D., Nachmani, G., & Rosenberg, S. Referent communication disturbances in acute schizophrenia. *Journal of Abnormal Psychology,* 1974, **83,** 1–13.

Connolly, K. J. & Bruner, J. S. *The growth of competence.* New York: Academic Press, 1974.

Corah, N. L., Anthony, E. J., Painter, P., Stern, J. A. & Thurston, D. Effects of perinatal anoxia after seven years. *Psychological Monographs,* 1965, **79,** 1–34.

Cowen, E. L., Pederson, A., Babigian, H., Izzo, L. D., & Trost, M. A. Long-term follow-up of early detected vulnerable children. *Journal of Consulting and Clinical Psychology,* 1973, **41,** 438–446.

Cromwell, R. L. & Wynne, L. C. The University of Rochester Child and Family Study: Development of competence and vulnerability in families at high-risk for schizophrenia. Rochester: mimeographed, 1974.

Dann, M., Levine, S. Z., & New, E. V. A long-term follow-up study of small premature infants. *Pediatrics,* 1964, **33,** 945–960.

Dohrenwend, B. P., Chin-Song, E. T., Egri, G., Mendelsohn, F. S., & Stokes, J. Measures of psychiatric disorder in contrasting class and ethnic groups (A preliminary report of ongoing research). In E. H. Hare and J. K. Wing (Eds.), *Psychiatric epidemiology.* New York: Oxford University Press, 1970, pp. 159–202.

Drillien, C. M. The incidence of mental and physical handicaps in school age children of very low birth weight. *Pediatrics,* 1961, **27,** 452–464.

Erlenmeyer-Kimling, L. Studies on the offspring of two schizophrenic parents. In D. Rosenthal and S. S. Kety (Eds.), *The transmission of schizophrenia.* New York: Pergamon Press, 1968, pp. 65–83.

Erlenmeyer-Kimling, L. Prospective study of schizophrenic parents. Progress Report, National Institute of Mental Health, 1974.

Erlenmeyer-Kimling, L. A prospective study of children at risk for schizophrenia: Methodological considerations and some preliminary findings. In R. D. Wirt, G. Winokur, and M. Roff (Eds.), *Life history research in psychopathology, Volume IV.* Minneapolis: University of Minnesota Press, 1975.

Ernhart, C. B., Graham, F. K., & Thurston, D. Relationship of neonatal apnea to development at three years. *Archives of Neurology,* 1960, **2,** 504–510.

Escalona, S. & Heider, G. M. *Prediction and outcome.* New York: Basic Books, 1959.

Fischer, M. Genetic and environmental factors in schizophrenia. *Acta Psychiatrica Scandinavica,* 1973, Supplement **238,** 158 pp.

Fish, B. & Hagin, R. Visual-motor disorders in infants at risk for schizophrenia. *Archives of General Psychiatry,* 1973, **28,** 900–904.

Fish, B., Wile, R., Shapiro, T., & Halpern, F. The prediction of schizophrenia in infancy. II. A ten-year follow-up report of predictions made at one month of age. In P. H. Hoch and J. Zubin (Eds.), *Psychopathology of schizophrenia.* New York: Grune and Stratton, 1966, pp. 335–353.

Garmezy, N. Competence and adaptation in adult schizophrenic patients and children at risk. In S. R. Dean (Ed.), *Schizophrenia: The first ten Dean award lectures.* New York: MSS Information Corporation, 1973, pp. 168–204.

Garmezy, N. Children at risk: The search for the antecedents of schizophrenia. Part II: Ongoing research programs, issues, and intervention. *Schizophrenia Bulletin,* 1974 (Summer), No. 9, 55–125.

Garmezy, N. & Nuechterlein, K. H. Invulnerable children: The fact and fiction of competence and disadvantage (Abstract). *American Journal of Orthopsychiatry,* 1972, **77,** 328–329.

Garmezy, N. & Streitman, S. Children at risk: The search for the antecedents of schizophrenia. Part I: Conceptual models and research methods. *Schizophrenia Bulletin,* 1974 (Spring), No. 8, 14–90.

Goldstein, M. J., Judd, L. L., Rodnick, E. H. Alkire, A., & Gould, E. A method for studying social influence and coping patterns within families of disturbed adolescents. *Journal of Nervous and Mental Disease,* 1968, **147,** 233–251.

Gottesman, I. I., & Shields, J. *Schizophrenia and genetics: A twin study vantage point.* New York: Academic Press, 1972.

Grunebaum, H., Weiss, J. L., Gallant, D., & Cohler, B. J. Attention in young children of psychotic mothers. *American Journal of Psychiatry,* 1974, **131,** 887–891.

Harmeling, J. D. & Jones, M. B. Birth weights of high school dropouts. *American Journal of Orthopsychiatry,* 1968, **38,** 63–66.

Heston, L. L. Psychiatric disorders in foster home reared children of schizophrenic mothers. *British Journal of Psychiatry,* 1966, **112,** 819–825.

Hollingshead, A. B. Two factor index of social position. Unpublished manuscript (mimeographed). Yale University, 1957.

Holzman, P. S., Proctor, L. R., Levy, D. L., Yasillow, N. J., Meltzer, H. Y., & Hurt, S. W. Eye-tracking dysfunctions in schizophrenic patients and their relatives. *Archives of General Psychiatry,* 1974, **31,** 143–154.

Jones, N. B. (Ed.). *Ethological studies of behavior.* Cambridge: Cambridge University Press, 1972.

Kagan, J. *Change and continuity in infancy.* New York: John Wiley, 1971.

Kagan, J., Rosman, B. L., Day, D., Albert, J., & Phillips, W. Information processing in the child: Significance of analytic and reflective attitudes. *Psychological Monographs,* 1964, **78,** 1, Whole No. 578.

Kaplan, A. *The conduct of inquiry.* San Francisco: Chandler, 1964.

Kety, S. S. Biochemical theories of schizophrenia. *Science,* 1959, **129,** 1528–1532, 1590–1596.

Kety, S. S. Biochemical hypotheses and studies. In L. Bellak and L. Loeb (Eds.), *The schizophrenic syndrome.* New York: Grune and Stratton, 1969, pp. 155–171.

Kety, S. S., Rosenthal, D., Schulsinger, F., & Wender, P. H. The types and prevalence of mental illness in the biological and adoptive families of adopted schizophrenics. *Journal of Psychiatric Research,* Supplement, 1968, 1: 345–362.

Kohn, M. L. Social class and schizophrenia: A critical review. In D. Rosenthal and S. S. Kety (Eds.), *The transmission of schizophrenia.* New York: Pergamon Press, 1968, pp. 155–173.

Lewis, M. & Rosenblum, L. A. (Eds.). *The effect of the infant on its caregiver.* New York: Wiley Interscience, 1974.

Lilienfeld, A. M., Pasamanick, B., & Rogers, M. Relationships between pregnancy experience and the development of certain neuropsychiatric disorders in childhood. *American Journal of Public Health,* 1955, **45,** 637–643.

Maher, B. *Principles of psychopathology.* New York: McGraw-Hill, 1966.

Marcus, J. Cerebral functioning in offspring of schizophrenics: A possible genetic factor. *International Journal of Mental Health,* 1974, **3,** 57–73.

Marcus, L. M. Studies of Attention in Children Vulnerable to Psychopathology. Unpublished Ph.D. dissertation. University of Minnesota, December, 1972.

McCord, W. & McCord, J. *Origins of crime.* New York: Columbia University Press, 1959.

McNeil, T. F. & Kaij, L. Obstetric complications and physical size of offspring of schizophrenic, schizophrenic-like, and control mothers. *British Journal of Psychiatry,* 1973, **123,** 341–348.

McNeil, T. F. & Kaij, L. Reproduction among female mental patients: Obstetric complications and physical size of offspring. *Acta Psychiatrica Scandinavica,* 1974, **50,** 3–15.

McNeil, T. F., Persson-Blennow, I., & Kaij, L. Reproduction in female psychiatric patients: Severity of mental disturbance near reproduction and rates of obstetric complications. *Acta Psychiatrica Scandinavica,* 1974, **50,** 23–32.

Mednick, S. A. & McNeil, T. F. Current methodology in research on the etiology of schizophrenia: Serious difficulties which suggest the use of the high-risk group method. *Psychological Bulletin,* 1968, **70,** 681–693.

Mednick, S. A., Mura, E., Schulsinger, F. & Mednick, B. Perinatal conditions and infant development in children with schizophrenic parents. *Social Biology,* 1971, **8,** S103–113.

Mednick, S. A. & Schulsinger, F. Some premorbid characteristics related to breakdown in children with schizophrenic mothers. In D. Rosenthal and S. S. Kety (Eds.), *The transmission of schizophrenia.* New York: Pergamon Press, 1968, pp. 267–291.

Mednick, S. & Schulsinger, F. Studies of children at high risk for schizophrenia. In S. R. Dean (Ed.), *Schizophrenia: The first ten Dean Award lectures.* New York: MSS Information Corporation, 1973, pp. 247–293.

Miller, D. Alternatives to mental patient rehospitalization. *Community Mental Health Journal,* 1966, **2,** 124–128.

Mizrahi, G. K., Mednick, S. A., Schulsinger, F., & Fuchs, F. Perinatal complications in children of schizophrenic mothers. *Acta Psychiatrica Scandinavica,* 1974, **50,** 553–568.

Murphy, D. L. & Wyatt, R. J. Reduced monoamine oxidase activity in blood platelets from schizophrenic patients. *Nature,* 1972, **238,** 225–226.

Neale, J. M. & Weintraub, S. Selecting variables for high-risk research. Position paper. Conference on Risk Research, Dorado Beach, Puerto Rico, October, 1972.

Nuechterlein, K. H. Competent disadvantaged children: A review of research. Unpublished summa cum laude thesis. University of Minnesota, 1970.

Pasamanick, B. & Knobloch, H. Epidemiological studies on the complications of pregnancy and the birth process. In G. Caplan (Ed.), *Prevention of mental disorders in children.* New York: Basic Books, 1961, pp. 74–94.

Pasaminick, B. & Knobloch, H. Retrospective studies on the epidemiology of reproductive causality: Old and new. *Merrill-Palmer Quarterly,* 1966, **12**, 7–26.

Rieder, R. O., Rosenthal, D., Wender, P., & Blumenthal, H. The offspring of schizophrenics: Fetal and neonatal deaths. *Archives of General Psychiatry,* 1975, **32**, 200–211.

Robins, L. N. *Deviant children grown up.* Baltimore: The Williams and Wilkins Company, 1966.

Rodnick, E. H. & Shakow, D., Set in the schizophrenic as measured by a composite reaction time index. *American Journal of Psychiatry,* 1940, **97**, 214–225.

Rolf, J. E. The academic and social competence of children vulnerable to schizophrenia and other behavior pathologies. *Journal of Abnormal Psychology,* 1972, **80**, 225–243.

Rolf, J. E. & Garmezy, N. The school performance of children vulnerable to behavior pathology. In D. Ricks, A. Thomas, and M. Roff (Eds.), *Life history research in psychopathology, Volume III.* Minneapolis: University of Minnesota Press, 1974, pp. 87–107.

Rolf, J. E. & Harig, P. T. Etiological research in schizophrenia and the rationale for primary prevention. *American Journal of Orthopsychiatry,* 1974, **44**, 538–554.

Rosenthal, D. (Ed.). *The genian quadruplets.* New York: Basic Books, 1963.

Rosenthal, D. A program of research on heredity in schizophrenia. *Behavioral Science,* 1971, **16**, 191–201.

Rosenthal, D. Evidence for a spectrum of schizophrenic disorders. Paper presented at the Annual Meeting of the American Psychological Association. New Orleans, Louisiana, August 31, 1974.

Rosenberg, S. & Cohen, B. D. Referential processes of speakers and listeners. *Psychological Review,* 1966, **73**, 208–231.

Sameroff, A. J. Infant risk factors in developmental deviancy. Paper presented at the meetings of the International Association for Child Psychiatry and Allied Professions. Philadelphia, July, 1974.

Sameroff, A. J. & Zax, M. Perinatal characteristics of the offspring of schizophrenic women. *Journal of Nervous and Mental Disease,* 1973a, **157**, 191–199.

Sameroff, A. J. & Zax, M. Schizotaxia revisited: Model issues in the etiology of schizophrenia. *American Journal of Orthopsychiatry,* 1973b, **43**, 744–754.

Schachter, J. The vulnerable child in infancy. Paper presented at the meetings of the International Association for Child Psychiatry and Allied Professions. Philadelphia, July, 1974.

Shea, M. J. A follow-up study into adulthood of adolescent psychiatric patients in relation to internalizing and externalizing symptoms, MMPI configurations, social competence and life history variables. Unpublished Ph.D. thesis, University of Minnesota, Minneapolis, 1972.

Smith, A. C., Flick, G. C., Ferriss, G. S. & Sellmann, A. H. Prediction of developmental outcome at seven years from prenatal, perinatal and postnatal events. *Child Development,* 1972, **43,** 495–507.

Sobel, D. E. The children of schizophrenic parents: Preliminary observation on early development. *American Journal of Psychiatry,* 1961, **118,** 512–517.

Strauss, J. S. & Carpenter, W. The prediction of outcome in schizophrenia: Part I. Characteristics of outcome. *Archives of General Psychiatry,* 1972, **27,** 739–746.

Strauss, J. S. & Carpenter, W. Characteristic symptoms and outcome in schizophrenia. *Archives of General Psychiatry,* 1974a, **30,** 429–434.

Strauss, J. S. & Carpenter, W. T. The prediction of outcome in schizophrenia: II. Relationships between predictor and outcome variables. *Archives of General Psychiatry,* 1974b, **31,** 37–42.

Thomas, A., Chess, S., & Birch, H. G. *Temperament and Behavior Disorders In Children.* New York: New York University Press, 1968.

Tinbergen, N. Foreward to *Ethological studies of behavior* (N. B. Jones, Ed.). Cambridge: Cambridge University Press, 1972.

Weintraub, S. A. Self-control as a correlate of an internalizing and externalizing symptom dimension. *Journal of Abnormal Child Psychology,* 1973, **1,** 292–307.

Wiener, G., Rider, R. V., Oppel, W. C., & Harper, P. A. Correlates of low birth weight: Psychological status at eight to ten years of age. *Pediatric Research,* 1968, **2,** 110–118.

Wyatt, R. J., Termini, B. A., & Davis, J. Biochemical and sleep studies of schizophrenia: A review of the literature. Part I. Biochemical studies. *Schizophrenia Bulletin,* 1971, No. 4, pp. 10–44.

Wynne, L. C. Strategies for sampling groups at high risk for the development of schizophrenia. Conference on Risk Research. National Institute of Mental Health, Bethesda, Maryland, June 12–13, 1969.

Yarrow, M. R., Campbell, J. D., & Burton, R. V. Recollections of childhood: A study of the retrospective method. *Monographs of the Society for Research in Child Development,* 1970, Serial No. 138, 35, (5).

Zubin, J. The biometric approach to psychopathology—revisited. In J. Zubin and C. Shagass (Eds.), *Neurobiological aspects of psychopathology.* New York: Grune and Stratton, 1969, pp. 281–309.

Zubin, J. Scientific models for psychopathology in the 1970's. In Scientific Models and Psychopathology (S. Fisher, Ed.). *Seminars in Psychiatry,* 1972, **4,** 283–296.

CHAPTER 6

Schizophrenia in Children of Schizophrenic Mothers*

SARNOFF A. MEDNICK, HANNE SCHULSINGER, AND FINI SCHULSINGER

In 1962 we began studying 207 children at high risk for schizophrenia (they have schizophrenic mothers). In the intervening years we have seen these individuals' lives follow a variety of courses; some have led rather "successful" lives, some have succumbed to a variety of mental disorders, and others have been repeatedly apprehended for criminal offenses. Our most recent examination of the sample (almost complete in November, 1974) included a rather thorough diagnostic interview. In this paper we describe the rationale and procedures of the high-risk method, some intermediate findings, the first results of the most recent diagnostic assessment, and a preliminary report of some premorbid characteristics of individuals who have become schizophrenic.

BACKGROUND CONSIDERATIONS

Depending on the age and the demographic and social structure of the reference population, one to three of every fifty children born will (at some time

*The research on the 1962 High-risk subjects is being supported by NIMH grant MH 25325. The most recent assessment of these subjects was supported by a grant from the Foundation for Child Development. The perinatal research is being supported by NIMH grant MH 19225.

The work in Mauritius is supported by the Mauritian Ministry of Health. We wish to express our gratitude to Sir Harold Walter and the government of Mauritius. The World Health Organization has supported the research with grants to the Psykologisk Institut of Copenhagen. The assessment of the 1800 children in Mauritius was supported by a grant from the British Medical Research Council to Peter Venables, and from the National Association for Mental Health to Brian Sutton-Smith. The Danish Organization for Aid to Developing Nations (DANIDA) supports the nursery schools.

217

in their lives) suffer a degree of schizophrenia sufficient to bring them to the attention of a psychiatric facility (Yolles & Kramer, 1969). Schizophrenia is the most serious of the mental illnesses. It most often strikes during young adulthood and can seriously disable the victim's life. Despite a variety of cross-national definitional difficulties these facts reflect the statistics observed in most or all developed countries. There is good reason to believe that schizophrenia is also observed in developing nations (Benedict, 1958); some evidence suggests that the prevalence of the condition is not radically different from that in the developed nations (Murphy & Raman, 1972).

Since its establishment as a diagnostic category eighty years ago, schizophrenia has attracted a rather impressive mass of research attention. Despite this, we have no inkling of its cause. One observer has rather dryly characterized the growing mountain of published material on schizophrenia as constituting an "independent problem of waste disposal."

Perhaps this paucity of research results exists to some large extent because investigators have largely restricted themselves to research designs exploring the correlates of *advanced* schizophrenia. For reasons that we will try to clarify, the correlative design is somewhat less than ideal for unearthing causes, especially in this area of investigation. We recommend, instead, the prevention model in which the advantages of the experimental-manipulative method may be exploited.

Since Kraepelin named the disorder dementia praecox, we have made no outstanding progress in our attempts to understand the details of its etiology. An exception to this is our recent increased understanding of the role of genetics in schizophrenia. This has not been due to a lack of interest or a lack of energetic effort. Nor has it been due to any understandable modesty concerning the consummation of pages of scientific journals. Quite the contrary. In contrast, the more "physical" illnesses of man seem to have yielded their secrets more readily. It may repay a moment's reflection to wonder why.

Research on etiology requires the construction of causative statements using the method of *experimental manipulation*. This is by far the method of choice in research on causes of disease. Thus we can inject a laboratory animal with a suspect virus and observe whether it develops a given illness. If it does, and we have used proper controls, we have unequivocally nailed down at least one partial cause. By analogy, to properly conduct experimental-manipulative research into the causes of schizophrenia we should systematically inflict children with those suspect life circumstances, biochemical and physiological anomalies that we hypothesize to be etiologically important and observe the outcome. Of course, we will not and cannot do this; the experimental-manipulative method is unavailable to us in this area.

On the other hand, for the bodily illnesses, organ systems sufficiently similar to those of humans may be found in laboratory animals. And so experimental-manipulative research can be done using these laboratory animals as subjects. However, the organ system under most serious suspicion in *mental* illness may not be sufficiently similar in man and the lower animals. There is, in any case, some uncertainty among most investigators that the so-called experimental or drug neuroses and psychoses that we can quickly induce in rats, cats, dogs, monkeys and man are in every, or any, way equivalent to a behavioral disturbance acquired by a human being over a period of many years.

To sum up, we believe that our poor progress relative to that of scientists studying the bodily illnesses is most likely not solely attributable to our greater stupidity, laziness, or scientific ineptitude. It is because our subjects are human and because their illnesses are peculiarly human that we are barred from using our most effective tools. Instead, we have done our best by constructing theories that are difficult to test truly and with elaborating the empirical correlates of schizophrenia.

But it is not our purpose either to find excuses for clinical research or to bury it, but rather to suggest viable alternatives. There *is* a way in which clinical research can exploit the efficiency and clarity of the experimental-manipulative method. The same humane code that inhibits us from experimentally manipulating the lives of children in attempts to cause them to become schizophrenic, would only encourage and support careful, well-founded attempts at experimental manipulations aimed at *preventing* mental illness. Let us hasten to make clear that even if such preventive attempts were effective, they would not point directly to etiology. Penicillin can cure or prevent an illness without giving us precise knowledge of causes. If, however, we administer vitamins to one group, and substitute-mothering experience to another, the relative success of these interventive procedures will suggest where we might most profitably search for causes.

The first step is the hardest. How are we to choose our methods of prevention so that we can get started? We approached this problem slowly and circumspectly. We are dealing with children whose lives should not be influenced in the absence of sufficient, research-tested grounds. Also, the effort and commitment involved in long-term prevention research is enormous.

What is there in the research literature that might suggest a reasonable preventive course for that single project? There are many sources that should be examined, but the primary one we sought was sound evidence related to etiology. Such evidence would immediately suggest hypotheses to be tested. We turned to an analysis of the research literature on schizophrenia.

This analysis has been published (Mednick & McNeil, 1968); we will spare the reader the joyless narrative of our disappointments. Briefly, we concluded that almost all the existing literature of schizophrenia has indeterminate relevance to the question of etiology or treatment. The research has studied the schizophrenic patient himself, his family, and school and clinical records he left behind as a child. These methods suffer from the disadvantage of beginning with an individual who is already schizophrenic. Studying the schizophrenic or his family tells us more about the consequences of being a schizophrenic than it does about the causes. The schizophrenic has suffered educational, economic, and social failure. He has experienced prehospital, hospital, and posthospital drug regimens; he tends to be a bachelor with little or no sexual experience. He is often tested after years of psychiatric institutionalization. He is overwhelmed by chronic illness, sheer unadulterated misery, or unending boredom. Controls for such experiences are not readily available; certainly the use of American college sophomores leaves one open to certain criticisms. *Consequences* of being schizophrenic (such as institutionalization) are in themselves quite sufficient to be completely responsible for some of the differences that have been reported between schizophrenic and control groups (Silverman et al., 1966). In effect, schizophrenics may be so contaminated by the consequences of their illness that they are not suitable subjects for research into the causes of their own illness.

Studies of the families of schizophrenics have been based on the often unexpressed "etiological assumption" that disturbed family processes have a role in the development of schizophrenia (Fontana, 1966). It is, however, just as reasonable to assume the obverse of this assumption: that the presence of a schizophrenic child or adolescent plays a role in the development of family disturbance. There is evidence for the latter assumption; studies of families of children with other severe chronic illnesses found them to be similar to families with schizophrenics. When high family conflict and maternal overprotection is reported for parents of diabetics (Crain et al., 1966a, 1966b), hemophiliacs (Mattson and Gross, 1966), infantile paralytics (Rosenbaum, 1943), and children with scoliosis and osteomyelitis (Kammerer, 1940), it seems likely that the conflict and overprotection are results rather than causes of the disease. (Note that we are *not* saying that this suggests that family variables are not involved in the etiology of schizophrenia. The study of families in which a member is already schizophrenic is simply not an excellent way to investigate this question).

A third approach is the childhood-records method, which analyses school, clinic, or birth records of schizophrenics. Although these records provide much useful information, there are serious drawbacks in their applicability for systematic research. The records were written by different teachers or therapists using different vocabularies; if one therapist calls a patient "nervous," is this equivalent to what another terms "tense"? And if a child is not labeled "nervous" does this mean he was not, or that the therapist merely did not mention it? When one works with records that are 20–30 years old there is no way to clarify these points. There are also serious problems in the differential migrancy rates of patients and potential controls (Mednick & McNeil, 1968, p. 686).

Because of these considerations we turned from the study of patients, to the longitudinal study of young children at high risk for schizophrenia, children who have chronically and severely schizophrenic mothers. In 1962, in Copenhagen, 207 such high-risk children as well as 104 controls were intensively examined. The controls had had no hospitalizations for mental illness in their families for three generations. The study is prospective and longitudinal (Mednick and Schulsinger, 1968). We intend to follow these 311 subjects for 20–25 years from our beginning date of 1962. During the course of these years we estimate that approximately 100 of the high-risk children will succumb to some form of mental illness; 25–30 should become schizophrenic (Kallmann, 1946; Heston, 1966).

Let us examine the strategy and logic of the high-risk design. It should be recalled that one great problem with previously discussed research was the absence of adequate controls. Figure 1 presents the design schematically. It can be conceptualized as developing at three levels. At the first level we have a cross-sectional comparison of 200 high-risk children and 100 matched low-risk children. At level II we can estimate from work by Heston (1966), Reisby (1967), and Kallmann (1946) that about 50% of the high-risk children will become seriously socially deviant. Rather good comparison subjects for these deviants are the nondeviant children with schizophrenic mothers and the low-risk controls. At the third level we can estimate that perhaps 30 of the 100 high-risk deviants will be diagnosed schizophrenic. An interesting set of controls for these schizophrenics are the 70 high-risk deviants, the 100 nondeviant high-risk children, and the low-risk children.

It is our intention to use information from this study in the design of prevention research. Because of this we must be especially concerned with the reliability of our findings. However, 25-year longitudinal studies are not readily replicated. Others using the same design may not be attracted to the same variables. In view of this, a form of replication was built into the design. At level II the 100 eventually deviant individuals can be conceived of as suffering breakdown in five waves of 20 subjects each. Thus, there are four potential replications of the first data analysis. The precision of the replications will of course be attenuated to the extent that the subsequent breakdown waves differ in age of diagnosis. The 30 schizophrenics can be conceived of as breaking down in two waves of 15 individuals each.

The high-risk design has certain advantages:

1.   The high-risk children when first examined have not yet experienced such aspects of the schizophrenic life as hospitalization or drugs. These factors

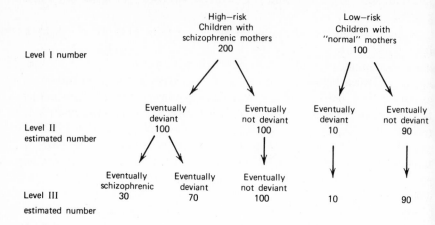

Figure 1.   Example of design of study of high-risk samples.

do not color their reactions to our test procedures.

2.   The researchers, relatives, teachers, and the subject himself do not know he will become schizophrenic. This relieves the data of a certain part of the burden of bias.

3.   The information we gather is relatively current. We can ask the high-risk adolescent or his family if he sees girls socially and how often. This is quite different from depending on the memory and cooperation of a 30-year-old schizophrenic patient or his 55-year-old mother.

4.   We obtain our data uniformly and systematically. For example, in this investigation we administered the Wechsler Intelligence Scale for Children. This was administered by the same examiner, using the same chairs, at the same table, in the same room, at the same time of day.

The long-term longitudinal study of children at high risk for schizophrenia is not without problems. The chief problem is maintaining contact with the subjects over a long period. It is in part for this reason that Denmark is an ideal location for such research. There is little emigration from Denmark; The Danish Folkeregister maintains at up-to-date register of the current address of every resident in Denmark. We can thus expect successful follow up of our subjects.

The fact that the high-risk children have at least one schizophrenic parent makes it difficult to consider their family-rearing conditions as representative. This is a serious problem; but since some portion of these children have been raised by nonschizophrenic foster parents or institutions, we have attempted to turn this situation to our advantage by the consideration of psychiatric outcome as a function of different family rearing conditions (Higgins, 1966).

Another serious difficulty that plagues longitudinal research is the danger that 20 years later one is stuck with measures that might then be considered dated and even trivial. We try to avoid this hazard by expanding and updating our initial experimental measures in subsequent follow-up examinations.

CHECK ON PSYCHIATRIC GENETICS LITERATURE

When we began in Copenhagen in 1962 it was clear to us that we were perhaps relying too heavily on reports from Germany and the United States that the probability of schizophrenia was relatively high among children with schizophrenic mothers. We determined to check these reports on a Danish sample selected in a manner that was almost identical to our own procedures. We supported the efforts of Dr. Niels Reisby in this study.

He began by finding the names of 98 female patients in four Danish mental hospitals. From the hospital records, the Folkeregister (an up-to-date record of the current address of every individual in Denmark), and the Institute of Psychiatric Demography, Aarhus Institute he prepared a list of their children. Again, at the Institute (where every psychiatric hospilization in Denmark is registered) he checked to see the percentage of these children that had been hospitalized for schizophrenia. This figure proved to be 12.7%. (He used Strömgren's modification of the Weinberg correction. The average age of the children was 34.8 years). The average age at first admission for those children who succumbed was 24.6 years. We can consider 12.7% to be a sizable underestimate of the prevalence of schizophrenia in this sample because well over 50% of these children live in rural areas of Denmark, but only 27% of those who were hospitalized for schizophrenia were from such farm areas. In terms of clinical experience and from surveys done in equivalent areas, it is known that the farm people shelter many harmless "trouble-free" schizophrenics and avoid hospitalization if at all possible. In any case, the figure 12.7% is not far from Kallmann's (1938) figure of 16%.

Of great interest in this study is the distribution of ages of the children at first admission (Table 1). In view of the fact that the mothers were selected in the same way as were the mothers in the current study, Table 1 has permitted us to estimate the rate at which schizophrenics would appear among the children of our sample. Thus, from Table 1 we estimated that approximately 50% of the expected schizophrenics would appear when the sample reached a mean age of 25 years in 1972; this estimate proved to be quite accurate.

Table 1.   Children with Schizophrenic Mothers[a]; Age of First Hospitalization for Mental Illness

Age	Percent
Below 20	38
21 – 25	14
26 – 30	10
31 – 35	24
36 – 40	10
41 and over	5

[a] The total number of cases is 21. The total number of mothers is 98. The mean age of the mothers at the time of investigation was 61.5 years; the children were 34.8 (from Reisby, 1967).

METHOD

Selection of Subjects

Parents of Groups

We chose to study children whose *mothers* are *process* schizophrenic for a number of reasons.(1) Allegations of paternity are not always free of challenge. It might be difficult to be quite sure of our major independent variable with alleged fathers, especially if they were schizophrenic. (2) Schizophrenic women have more children than schizophrenic men (Goldfarb & Erlenmeyer-Kimling, 1962). In a study of all schizophrenic men in a Danish state hospital we found schizophrenic women to be five times as fertile as schizophrenic men. (3) Psychodevelopmentally, mothers presumably play a greater role in shaping children. Using mothers has permitted us to carry out research on the effects of being reared by a schizophrenic mother (Higgins, 1966). (4) The offspring of process (typical schizophrenic) mothers yielded a higher rate of schizophrenia (Schulz, 1939, 1940: Lewis, 1957).

Diagnosis of Mother

Two experienced Danish psychiatrists trained together and then independently tested their reliability in making judgements from hospital records. Their agreement as to diagnosis on 20 test cases was found to be 100%. They merely had to judge whether the mothers were typical schizophrenics. They were instructed to discard *any* questionable cases. Following this reliability check, only one psychiatrist checked each record. For each mother a precoded form was filled out which listed her symptoms, provided information concerning her dates of hospitalization, and made a summary of her clinical status.

The intent in the selection of the mothers was to choose only cases that would be readily agreed upon in Europe or the United States as being severe and typical schizophrenics. We required at least 5 years of hospitalization, or at least three separate periods of hospitalization, each of at least 3 months' duration, with no sign of remission during discharge, or an extended hospitalization plus a certified State Invalid Pension for schizophrenia. Excluded were cases that did not have at least two different types of severe schizophrenic symptoms.

Matching of High-Risk and Low-Risk Subjects.

Pairs of high-risk (H) subjects were matched on sex, age, father's occupation (the best measure of social class in Denmark; Svalastoga, 1959), rural–urban residence, years of education, and institutional upbringing versus family life. Next, a single low-risk (L) subject was selected who was matched on these same variables individual for individual with each H pair.

In the case where an H child was in a children's home, he would be paired with another H child in a children's home. L children were also sampled from children's homes. They afford the opportunity of some degree of control for the broken-home aspects of being a child of a schizophrenic mother. This matching for children's home status had an interesting, unforeseen, but fortunate consequence. L subjects were not permitted to have had a mental illness that resulted in hospitalization in themselves, their parents or grandparents. The two major reasons for children being sent to a children's home were either serious mental illness or criminality in the parents. Since we screened for mental illness, the L group ended up with an unusual number of criminals among the fathers. Over 55% are known to the police while 42% have one or more convictions. Since schizophrenic women and criminal men mate assortatively (Kirkegaard-Sorensen & Mednick, 1975) the fathers of the H group match the L group fathers very well for degree of criminality. By our decision of taking L group children from institutions we accidentally matched L and H fathers for level of criminality. This has shown itself to be an important variable in understanding life outcome and individual characteristics of the children.

Table 2 presents the mean values for the H and L groups for the matching variable used in this study. As may be seen, the average age of the sample was 15.1 years at the time of the initial testing (1962). There would have been some advantage in testing a younger group; however, the average subject will not pass through the major risk period for schizophrenia before 1987. The subjects' mean age was selected so as to maximize the probability that the principal investigators would still be alive at the conclusion of this risk period. Studies of 3-years-old (Bell et al., in press; Schulsinger et al., in press) and 11-year-old high-risk samples (Mednick et al., 1971) have also been undertaken, but not with identical risk factors.

Table 2.   Characteristics of the Experimental and Control Samples

	Control	Experimental
Number of cases	104	207
Number of boys	59	121
Number of girls	45	86
Mean age[a]	15.1	15.1
Mean social class[b]	2.3	2.2
Mean years education	7.3	7.0
Percent of group in children's homes (5 years or more)[c]	14%	16%
Mean number of years in children's homes (5 years or more)[c]	8.5	9.4
Percent of group with rural residence[d]	22%	26%

[a] Defined as age to the nearest whole year.

[b] The scale runs from 0 (low) to 6 (high) and was adapted from Svalastoga (1959).

[c] We only considered experience in children's homes of 5 years or greater duration. Many of the Experimental children had been to children's homes for brief periods while their mothers were hospitalized. These experiences were seen as quite different from the experience of children who actually had to make a children's home their home until they could go out and earn their own living.

[d] A rural residence was defined as living in a town with a population of 2500 persons or fewer.

Alarm Network

As the subjects of the long-term follow up begin to breakdown, it will be crucial to be on the spot as soon as possible in order to gain a picture of the circumstances precipitating the breakdown. An alarm network was instituted to deal with this problem. First, through the health insurance system, each of the subjects has a family physician. These physicians are alerted to the fact that their patients are under study and provide information concerning contacts they may have with the subjects.

All hospitals on Zealand and all psychiatric hospitals in Denmark have submitted blank hospital registration cards to us. The 311 subjects have had these registration cards prepared for them using the particular forms of cards for each hospital. Also stamped on each card is a message requesting that the project be informed immediately if the subject presents himself for hospitalization. The secretaries responsible for informing us receive small financial incentives for every notification. The network has been operative for 10 years and seems highly effective. In addition to this, regular checks are made in the Psychiatric Register of the Demographic Institute.

Procedures

Until testing was complete none of the examiners was informed regarding whether the children tested were H or L subjects. All visits were scheduled by the social worker. The procedures were identical for all subjects.

In addition to weight and height the following measures were taken in the intensive 1962 examinations:

1. Psychophysiological conditioning and extinction testing.
2. Wechsler Intelligence Scale for Children (Danish adaptation).
3. Personality Inventory.
4. Word Association Test.
5. Continous Association Test.
6. Adjective Check List.
7. Psychiatric interview, yielding level of adjustment rating.
8. Parent interview.
9. School report.
10. Midwife's report on pregnancy and delivery.

RESULTS

As of 1967, the first wave of 20 breakdowns (which we call the sick group) had been identified. (For their clinical status see Table 3.) Of these, 13 had been admitted to psychiatric hospitals or had received psychological treatment. They had been given many diagnoses including schizophrenia. The seven not admitted included some who were probably schizophrenic. The clinical status of these individuals was ascertained by our follow up procedures. To each of these 20 we matched another high-risk subject(well group) of the same age, sex, social class, and institutional rearing status. In addition we matched these subjects for the psychiatrist's 1962 level of adjustment rating. We tried as much as possible to select for the well group individuals who, since 1962, had shown some improvement in level of adjustment. Also 20 individuals selected from the low-risk group constituted a control group for comparison purposes.

This matching yielded two groups of high-risk subjects. In 1962, both were judged to be equal in level of adjustment. Yet since then, one group has improved in level of mental health; the other group has suffered psychiatric breakdown. Why? Part of the answer could lie with the predisposing characteristics measured in 1962 at the time of the intensive examination.

The most important characteristics distinguishing the Sick Group from the Well and Control Group were the following:

Table 3.   Descriptions of Conditions of Sick Group

Male, born 16 March 1953; extremely withdrawn, no close contacts, 2 months' psychiatric admission following theft, currently in institution for boys with behavior difficulties, still performing petty thieveries.

Female, born 19 January 1943; married, one child, extremely withdrawn, nervous. Evidence of delusional thinking, pulls her hair out, has large bald area.

Female, born 29 March 1946; promiscuous, highly unstable in work, no close contacts, confused and unrealistic, psychiatric admission for diagnostic reasons, recent abortion, some evidence of thought disorder.

Male, born 1 July 1946; under minor provocation had had semipsychotic breakdown in Army, expresses strange distortions of his body image, thought processes vague, immature.

Male, born 2 May 1944; severe difficulties in concentrating; cannot complete tasks; marked schizoid character; marginally adjusted.

Male, born 3 June 1947; lonely in the extreme; spends all spare time at home; manages at home only by virtue of extremely compulsive routines; no heterosexual activity; marked schizoid character.

Male born 1 October 1953; no close contact with peers, attends class for retarded children, abuses younger children, recently took a little boy out in the forest, undressed him, urinated on him and his clothes, and sent him home.

Male, born 17 January 1954; has history of convulsions, constantly takes antiseizure drug (Dilanthin), nervous, confabulating, unhappy, sees frightening "nightmares" during the day; afraid of going to sleep because of nightmares and fear that people are watching through the window, feels teacher punishes him unjustly.

Female, born 18 March 1944; nervous quick mood changes; body image distortions, passive, resigned; psychiatric admission, paranoid tendencies revealed, vague train of thought.

Male, born 14 March 1952; arrested for involvement in theft of motorbike; extremely withdrawn, difficulties in concentration; passive, disinterested, father objected to his being institutionalized; consequently he is now out under psychiatric supervision.

Male, born 19 October 1947; level of intellectual performance in apprenticeship decreasing, private life extremely disorderly; abreacts through alcoholism.

Male, born 20 January 1944; severe schizoid character, no heterosexual activity; lives an immature, shy, anhedonic life, thought disturbances revealed in TAT.

Female, born 25 May 1947; psychiatric admission, abortion, hospital report suspects pseudoneurotic or early schizophrenia; association tests betray thought disturbance, tense, guarded, ambivalent. Current difficulties somewhat precipitated by sudden death of boy friend.

Male, born 13 August 1950; sensitive, negativistic, unrealistic; recently stopped working and was referred to a youth guidance clinic for evaluation. Is now under regular supervision of a psychologist.

Male, born 28 May 1947; history of car stealing, unstable, drifting, unemployed, sensitive, easily hurt, one year institutionalization in a reformatory for the worst delinquents in Denmark.

Female, born 1 June 1945; psychotic episode, one year of hospitalization; diagnoses from 2 hospitals; (1) schizophrenia, (2) manic psychosis.

Male, born 3 September 1946; severe schizoid character; psychotic breakdown in Army, preceded by arrest for car thievery. Now hospitalized.

Male, born 28 January 1953; perhaps border-line retarded; psychiatric admission for diagnostic reasons; spells of uncontrolled behavior.

Male, born 23 June 1948; repeatedly apprehended for stealing; severe mood swings, sensitive, restless, unrealistic; fired from job because of financial irregularities.

Female, born 5 July 1941; highly intelligent girl with mystical interests. Very much afflicted by mother's schizophrenia. TAT reveals thought disorder. Receiving psychotherapy.

1.   Those in the sick group lost their schizophrenic mothers to psychiatric hospitalization much earlier in their lives than did the other two groups. These

early-hospitalized mothers were also more severely schizophrenic. Individuals in the well group lost their mothers at approximately the same time as did the control group. In view of the greater severity of illness of the mothers who left their homes early, these data may be interpreted in relatively genetic or environmental terms.

2.   The teachers' reports indicated that the subjects in the sick group tended to be disturbing to the class. They were disciplinary problems and tended to be domineering and aggressive. They created conflicts and disrupted the class with their talking. This was true of 53% of the sick group, 18% of the well group, and 11% of the control group.

3.   On the Continual Association Test, where the subject is asked to give in one minute as many single-word associations as he can to a stimulus word, the sick group showed two distinctive patterns. These individuals had a strong tendency to rattle off a whole series words that were interrelated but, contextually, relatively irrelevant. Their associations also tended to "drift" away from the stimulus work. Contrary to instructions and cautions they might begin responding to their own responses; for example, to the stimulus word "table" they might respond "chair, top, leg, girl, pretty, sky . . . ". Those in the sick group who do not show drifting can apparently manage to avoid this only by restricting themselves to one or two responses per stimulus word for the entire one-minute period.

4.   Some of the variables most sharply differentiating the sick group from the well and control groups were electrodermal measures (GSR) taken during the psychophysiological testing. These measures largely reflect the functioning of the body's stress mobilization mechanisms.

a)   The latency of the GSR was substantially shorter for the sick group than for either of the other two groups.

b)   The GSR latency for the sick group did not show any signs of habituation. This was especially marked in the responses to the UCS (unconditioned stimulus) stress stimulus trials. The control and well groups' rapid habituation of latency was seen in the progressive increase of their response latencies from the first to the last of the stress trials. The latencies of the sick group, on the other hand, progressively decreased, suggesting a negative habituation or even increasing irritability. From the first to the last UCS trial, 69% of the well group exhibited a slowing of response latency (habituation); 75% of the sick group actually *increased* the speed of their response.

c)   A well-documented characteristic of conditioned GSR behavior is the rapidity with which it demonstrates experimental extinction. In both the well and the control groups electrodermal responsiveness was already dropping off by the end of the stress stimulus trials. After these stress trials we presented a series of nine nonreinforced test trials for generalization and speed of extinction of the conditioned response. The well and control groups displayed very rapid extinction; that is, they responded to only one or two of the extinction test trials. The sick group, however, exhibited great resistance to extinction, in many cases, responding with tenacity until the very end of the extinction series.

d)   The sick group showed a remarkably fast rate of recovery from momentary states of automatic imbalance. Once a GSR was made, we measured the rate at which recovery to basal level proceeded. On some trials rate of recovery almost perfectly separated the sick and control groups. The pooled sick and well groups' distributions for rate of recovery typically found 70% of the sick and 30% of the well group above the median.

The above material is discussed in greater detail in Mednick and Schulsinger (1968).

5.   In a previous report on the differences between the sick, well, and control groups we pointed out that, although in our analyses of data on birth complications "there was a slight general tendency for the sick group to have had a more difficult birth, none of the differences reached statistical significance" (Mednick & Schulsinger, 1968, pp. 280–281). Subsequent, more careful, examination of these data revealed, however, that although it was true that no single complication significantly differentiated the groups, 70% of the members of the sick group had suffered one or more serious pregnancy or birth complications (PBC). This contrasted with 15% of the well group and 33% of the control group. The PBCs included anoxia, prematurity, prolonged labor, placental difficulty, umbilical cord complications, mother's illness during pregnancy, multiple births, and breech presentations. Careful perusal of these data brought out an additional striking relationship within the sick group; there was a marked correspondence between PBCs and the anomalous electrodermal behavior reported above. Much of the GSR differences between the sick and well groups could be explained by the PBCs in the sick group. In the control group and low-risk group the PBCs were not as strongly associated with these extreme GSR effects. This suggests that the PBCs trigger some characteristics that may be genetically predisposed.

In a rather speculative article on the possible role of hippocampal dysfunction in schizophrenia, Mednick (1970) compared the distinguishing characteristics of the sick group with the characteristics reported for hippocampectomized rats.

Both the sick group subjects with PBCs and the hippocampal rats manifest fast response latency, very poor habituation, and poor extinction of a conditioned response. We can also tentatively link the hyperactivity of the hippocampal rats to the unruly classroom behavior of our Sick Group subjects. The two points that do not immediately relate to each other are the fast avoidance conditioning of the hippocampal rats and the fast GSR recovery of the sick group with PBCs (Mednick, 1970, p. 58).

The "hippocampus" hypothesis has received both support (McLardy, 1973a, 1973b, Bagshaw & Kimble, 1972) and criticism (Kessler & Neale, 1974) in the literature. But for our purposes the critical aspect is the attempt made in the article to link functionally the characteristics of fast autonomic recovery and fast avoidance conditioning. This linking contains the essence of a microtheory of how one becomes schizophrenic.

A MICROTHEORY OF SCHIZOPHRENIA

As stated in a more clinical formulation of the theory (Mednick, 1962), schizophrenia is an evasion of life and this evasion is learned. The learning, it is suggested, takes place gradually over a period of years. It is this learning of evasion or avoidance, on the basis of physiological aptitude, which comprises an important part of the clinical syndrome, schizophrenia.

To understand the importance of recovery to this theory we must first clarify our view of avoidance learning. Consider the rat in the shuttle box. The rat is first placed in compartment A, a bell rings, Ten seconds later the floor of compartment A is electrified. The rat leaps up, runs around, defecates, urinates, and eventually runs into B and safety. After perhaps 10 trials, the rat will learn to avoid the shock by running into B at the sound of the bell. It is important to ask the question, "What factors are important in producing this avoidance learning in the rat?" An obvious and critical factor is that he has a response of fear to the shock and bell. The greater the fear, the faster his learning to avoid. Another critical but perhaps less obvious factor is that when the rat runs into the safe compartment, he is rewarded by fear reduction. To be more precise, his avoidance response is rewarded by fear reduction. The value of a reinforcement is directly related to its speed of delivery and magnitude. The faster and greater the reduction of fear, the greater the reinforcement value. The rate at which this fear is reduced depends in large part on the rate at which the autonomic nervous system recovers from a fear state to a normal level. The faster the rate of recovery, the faster the delivery of the reinforcement and the greater the reinforcement. If the rat recovers very slowly, the difference between the shock compartment and the safe compartment will be minimized as will be the reinforcement value of his avoidance response. If the rat has abnormally fast autonomic recovery his reinforcement will come abnormally quickly; he will learn the avoidance response abnormally quickly. Hyperresponsiveness (and poor habituation and quick latency) and fast autonomic recovery, then, function as aptitudes for learning avoidance responses just as nimble fingers and absolute pitch provide aptitudes for learning to play the violin.

A human does not have to run to avoid an anxiety-producing stimulus. He can learn to avoid with situationally irrelevant thoughts. These irrelevant thoughts will take him from an anxiety-producing stimulus. If he has fast recovery, the thoughts will be rewarded and will increase in their probability of being elicited in the presence of anxiety. Over years, the pre-schizophrenic will learn more and more of these avoidant thoughts. When his thinking is predominantly evasive, a clinician will be able to note the thought disorder and will diagnose schizophrenia. Note that this formulation requires not only the ANS deviance but also a noxious environment.

Our theory suggests that the combination of:

1. An autonomic nervous system that responds too quickly and too much (and habituates poorly); and
2. an abnormally fast rate of recovery,

provide an aptitude for learning avoidance responses. These ANS variables may be profitably classified into two categories, those that can produce ANS distress (fast latency, exaggerated response amplitude, and lack of habituation) and the variable (fast recovery) that helps resolve the distress by providing an aptitude for learning to avoid distressing stimuli. If an individual is to become schizophrenic he must possess both of the types of ANS characteristics. If an individual is rapidly, exaggeratedly, and untiringly emotionally reactive he may become anxious or psychotic, but will not tend to learn schizophrenia unless his rate of recovery tends to be very fast. It also seems likely that an extraordinarily reactive ANS will only require moderately fast recovery while an extraordinarily fast recovery will only require moderate reactivity. Both very high reactivity and very fast recovery will result in a very heavy predisposition for schizophrenia.

We have stressed the importance of the physiological predispositions. But the hypothesized ANS predispositions will only result in distress in *response* to unpleasant environments or noxious thoughts. An individual who is treated kindly is far less likely to evidence distressing ANS overexcitement and will have relatively little provocation to learn a massive pattern of avoidant responses. The development of schizophrenia depends then on an interaction of reactive, sensitive, and quickly recovering autonomic nervous systems and unkind environments.

Empirical Evidence Concerning "Recovery" Microtheory

This theoretical orientation singles out autonomic recovery as a critical etiological factor in schizophrenia. It would seem relatively straightforward to test this hypothesis by simply measuring autonomic recovery. It is difficult, however, to measure autonomic functioning directly; most investigators content themselves with peripheral measures such as heart rate, blood pressure, respiration, and skin conductance. Since these measures do not always intercorrelate satisfactorily it is difficult to readily support the notion that all of these peripheral effects reflect central autonomic functioning. In view of this, research results with any single peripheral measure of autonomic activity cannot be used as unequivocal support or as an unequivocal criticism of the theory.

However, changes in the customary peripheral measures of autonomic functioning are probably not *totally* unrelated to central autonomic changes. Consequently, despite these cautions, if any single peripheral measure indicates that an individual evidences a pattern of fast recovery, such evidence should most likely *not* be seen as a basis for rejecting the hypothesis that his autonomic nervous system recovers quickly.

In this context we can briefly consider the evidence available concerning peripheral measures of recovery of autonomic functioning. The reader is referred to Mednick (1974) and Venables (1974) for more complete treatment of this material.

While the galvanic skin response and the electrodermal response (EDR) have interested psychologists and physiologists for some time, it is only relatively recently (and relatively infrequently) that they have attended systematically to the manner in which the function returns to its resting level. As Furedy (1972) indicates, electrodermal recovery (EDRec) is an "important but relatively ignored, characteristic of electrodermal behaviour" (p. 282). Darrow (1937) and Freeman and Katzoff (1942) published statements on recovery and in 1958 Mednick gave this variable a central role in a theory of schizophrenia. He hypothesized that preschizophrenics would be characterized by slow autonomic nervous system recovery.

This hypothesis was rejected in 1964 when Mednick and Schulsinger observed that the EDRec of their high-risk subjects was substantially faster than that of controls. As mentioned above, this finding was strongly supported by the results for the sick group. If EDRec is significantly related to the process of schizophrenia, and is not altered by the schizophrenic process or its consequents (e.g., hospitalization), then one would expect to observe fast EDRec in individuals already schizophrenic. Ax and Bamford (1970), reanalyzing taped EDRec data, found faster EDRec in chronic schizophrenics than in well-selected controls. Gruzelier and Venables (1972) and Gruzelier (1973) also reported faster EDRec for schizophrenics than for controls. In an investigation just completed in Venables's laboratory this fast EDRec finding for schizophrenics has again been confirmed (Venables, personal communication). In a paper in press, Janes and Stern have studied a recovery-related skin potential measure with high-risk children and controls rated for level of adjustement. Their findings support the hypothesis of faster recovery for the disturbed subjects. This finding with another peripheral measure of autonomic recovery does not yet cause us to reject the possibility that the skin conductance and skin potential findings are both reflecting some central autonomic process.

Garmezy (1974) has reported the results of an umpublished study by Erlenmeyer-Kimling and Rainer. In this study they tested recovery in 34 high-risk children (7–12 years of age) and 23 controls. All of these children came from intact families. No differences were found between the groups in recovery. We have two comments. As will be described in detail below, in our most recent diagnostic examination the interviewer diagnosed 14 schizophrenics among our high-risk subjects. We checked to see how many might have been rejected by Erlenmeyer-Kimling and Rainer because of lack of intact family. Twelve of the 14 would have been rejected. Thus we must ask how many future schizophrenics are included in the 34 risk subjects tested by Erlenmeyer-Kimling and Rainer. One might even ask what special strengths the parents of the high-risk children must have to maintain an intact family in the face of schizophrenia in one or both spouses. We reanalyzed our recovery data taking only families that would meet Erlenmeyer-Kimling and Rainer's criterion of intactness. This group is a small minority of the high-risk group. Our findings for this "intact" subgroup are consonant with Erlenmeyer-Kimling and Rainer's.

An unpublished study by Van Dyke investigated EDRec in adult adoptees who had a schizophrenic biological parent. He found no significant differences in EDRec between the high-risk and low-risk subjects. This study was completed at the Psykologisk Institut in Copenhagen. When we first learned of Van Dyke's results we immediately suspected the reason for the disparate results. As pointed out above, schizophrenics tend to mate assortatively with criminals (Kirkegaard-Sorensen & Mednick, 1975). Criminals tend to exhibit exceptionally slow autonomic recovery (Bader-Bartfai, 1974; Hare, personal communication; Mednick et al., 1974; Mednick & Loeb, unpublished manuscript, 1974). In a twin study at our laboratory in Copenhagen we have found evidence that EDRec has a strong genetic component. In our longitudinal studies, children of criminals and psychopaths evidence markedly slow EDRec.

All of these facts suggested to us that perhaps Van Dyke's high-risk subjects and their fathers were more criminal than the low-risk children and their fathers. This would result in a slowing of the EDRec measured in the high-risk children. Since the data were available to us in Copenhagen, with the cooperation of Drs. Rosenthal and Van Dyke, we checked the criminality in the high-and low-risk children and their fathers. Indeed, as predicted, the level of criminality was considerably higher in the high-risk group for number of months in jail (mean for high-risk fathers = 4.73 months; mean for low-risk fathers = 1.84 months). It seems possible that part of the reason Van Dyke failed to find EDRec differences between his high-and low-risk subjects was the relatively high level of criminality in his high-risk group.

In four independent laboratories in three nations, evidence has been reported supporting the hypothesis that preschizophrenics and schizophrenics are characterized by fast EDRec. In one of these instances the peripheral autonomic measure was skin potential. In the other studies the autonomic measure was skin conductance. These data do not encourage us to reject the hypothesis that preschizophrenics and schizophrenics are characterized by abnormally fast recovery of the autonomic nervous system.

Hippocampal Functioning and Recovery

We indicated above that speculations have been advanced implicating hippocampal disfunction in the etiology of schizophrenia (Mednick, 1970). In support of this, literature was cited which pointed to the similarity in symptoms of schizophrenia and psychomotor epilepsy. These disorders often require very careful examination before a reliable differential diagnosis can be achieved. They do have different causes and prognoses, but psychomotor epileptics have been mistakenly diagnosed as schizophrenics. A recent study by Novelly, Graham, and Ax (1974) has compared psychomotor epileptics, normal controls, and schizophrenics on a number of psychophysiological measures including EDRec. The schizophrenics and the psychomotor epileptics resembled each other closely on all the measures but one, EDRec. The schizophrenics showed faster EDRec than the psychomotor epileptics and the normal controls. This finding emphasizes the apparent specificity of fast EDRec for schizophrenia.

Avoidance Learning and Schizophrenia.

Our theoretical orientation would predict faster avoidance conditioning for schizophrenics than nonschizophrenics. An effective measure of avoidance conditioning with humans is eyelid conditioning. The task here is to learn to close an eyelid to a warning signal in order to avoid the noxious effects of a puff of air on the eyeball. Workers in this field can distinguish between voluntary, involuntary, and conditioned blinks. Spain (1966) demonstrated that schizophrenics learn this avoidance response *faster than normals*. In addition those schizophrenics that evidenced the most withdrawn (avoidant) ward behaviour manifested the fastest avoidance conditioning.

We would also expect relatively good performance from schizophrenics in situations where learning of an avoidance response is functional. In general, censure or punishment produces marked deterioration in schizophrenics' performance (Rodnick & Garmezy, 1957). If, however, the situation is constructed so that the schizophrenic can learn to avoid the censure, his performance improves disproportionately (Cavanaugh, 1958; Losen, 1961; Johannesen, 1964). Unlike normal subjects, schizophrenics learn faster when their response can avoid punishment than when their response merely produces reward (Atkinson & Robinson, 1961).

In our own high-risk sample we would predict that those with fast recovery will have learned more avoidant associates. In a test of this hypothesis in the 1967 breakdown subjects and their controls Lampasso has found a positive correlation between recovery rate and a score for avoidant word associations ($r = .48$, 25 df, $p < .05$).

Results of 1972 Diagnostic Assessment

As pointed out above, the Reisby (1967) study gave us reason to expect that when the sample had reached an average age of 25 we should expect to be able to diagnose approximately half of the eventual schizophrenics in the high-risk group. Following the logic of our design (see Figure 1) we initiated an intensive assessment of the high- and low-risk samples in 1972 when they reached an average age of 25.1 years. (They ranged between 20 and 30 years of age). The important goal of this reassessment was the establishment of a reliable diagnosis and an evaluation of their current life status. This assessment included psychophysiological and cognitive tests, a social interview, and a battery of diagnostic devices. The diagnostic devices included a 3¼-hour clinical interview by an experienced diagnostician, a full MMPI, providing an independent objective diagnosis, and the possible psychiatric hospitalization diagnoses and records. The diagnostician completed the Endicott and Spitzer, *Current and Past Psychopathology Scales* (CAPPS) (1972) and the *Wing Present Status Examination* (PSE) 9th edition (Wing, Cooper and Sartorius, 1974). Both of these scales yield computer-derived diagnoses. The clinician also made a clinical diagnosis. It should be pointed out that the interview also contained scales evaluating thought structure and disorder, intellectual functioning, motoric functioning, ego-organization, ego-identity, ego-maturity, emotional contact, neurosis, schizoid personality, psychopathy, organic traits, and positive traits and appearance.

Interview Procedures

Training

The interviewer was trained in London in John Wing's department in the use of the PSE until she reached satisfactory levels of reliability. She received instruction in the use of the CAPPS in New York from Endicott and Spitzer.

Interview Construction

The interview was structured as a clinical procedure, not as a questionnaire.

There was a reliance on open questions so that the subject had the opportunity to express himself spontaneously. At the same time, it was necessary for the interview to cover a certain amount of ground in terms of the demands of the various scales in the interview. Thus the interviewer sought a balance between the more structured and the more open-ended aspects of the interview. An additional consideration was the maintenance of excellent rapport between the project and the subject to assure his future cooperation.

Choice of CAPPS and PSE

These computer-scored interviews were used in order to facilitate communication internationally regarding the diagnostic labels we affix to the subjects. We were also attracted by the reliability of the instruments. The PSE has the advantage of being based on a traditional, conservative diagnostic assessment sensitive to signs of schizophrenia expressed during the interview and in the past month. The PSE also derives an index of "caseness" which indicates on a scale of 1–9 how much the interviewee resembles a psychiatric case. This may be seen as an index of seriousness of psychiatric illness. Such an index is especially useful in studies of nonpatient samples such as are described in this paper. It should be pointed out that the index is in the process of being developed by John Wing. Results used in this report are not final; the final version will be published after more extensive testing.

The CAPPS contains an anamnestic section that supplements the PSE current status emphasis. The CAPPS, having been constructed in accordance with broader United States diagnostic definitions, was expected to be less conservative than the clinical diagnosis that followed a Scandinavian narrow definition. The CAPPS also yields factor analysis derived scales relating to social and psychological aspects of the interviewee's development.

Because the PSE is intended to describe only the current status of the interviewee it was expected that individuals who had suffered a schizophrenic episode more than a month before the interview but who currently were in good remission would not be classified schizophrenic.*

Course of Interview

When the subject arrived at 8:30 a.m. the interviewer was blind to his high- or low-risk status. She administered the PSE and items from the CAPPS current scales. The interview was audio taped in view of the subject. The PSE and CAPPS current scale took 1½ hours. After this the subject went to other parts of the testing program.

The interviewer then recorded answers to the PSE and CAPPS current scale

---

*The Syndrome Checklist for previous episodes, and the Aetiology Schedule, were not used at this stage of the investigation.

and wrote a summary of the subject's behavior, attitude, symptoms, i.e., the clinical impression the subject had made. A tentative diagnosis was also made at this point. The interviewer then was informed of the group status of the subject and supplied with all of the information present in the subject's file. The interviewer read this material and wrote a summary.

In the afternoon, the subject returned for an additional 1¾-hours of interview. This covered the CAPPS historical sections and the various scales of the clinical interview. Items of the CAPPS relating to social and occupational functioning were completed by the social worker during a home visit with the subject.

At the conclusion of the interview the interviewer prepared a final summary of the life history of the subject and made a diagnosis. The World Health Organization International Classification of Disorders (1967) was the framework of the diagnosis.

The coded PSE and CAPPS materials were sent to London and New York, respectively; computer diagnoses were returned.* In all we will be able to compare five diagnostic sources, possible hospital diagnosis, PSE Catego diagnosis, CAPPS diagnosis, clinical diagnosis, and MMPI diagnosis. (Professor Irving Gottesman is independently preparing the MMPI diagnoses). In this paper we will report on the PSE, CAPPS, and clinical diagnoses.

Subjects

Table 4 presents information on the results of our contacts with the subjects. As can be seen there are eight of the high-risk subjects who died in the course of these 10 years; none of the low-risk subjects have died. This is a dramatic difference. Of the eight, six died before the assessments began. The other two took part in the assessment. Thus at the beginning of the assessment 201 high-risk subjects were available. Of these, 173 took part only in the full interview; 10 took part in the home interview by the social worker. Thus 91% have taken some part in the interview. The social worker (who has known these subjects for the past 12 years) is confident that many of the remaining subjects will be in for interview when they return from abroad or when special personal circumstances are altered. Of the low-risk subjects, 91 took part in the full interview; six took part only in the home interview. Thus 93% of the low-risk group has taken some part in the interview.

Table 5 presents identifying information on those who completed the full interview. The groups are well matched with each other and with the total

*We wish to acknowledge the kindness of Professor John K. Wing and Drs. Jean Endicott and Robert Spitzer for their aid in utilizing their interview materials and for scoring the resultant protocols.

Table 4. Followup Results with 1962 Samples

	High Risk (N=207)	Low Risk (N=104)
Full assessment complete	173	91
Home interview only (social worker)	10	6
Not yet contacted[a]	6	2
(Parent objected or the subject could not be located)		
Living abroad[a]	4	0
Deceased[b]	8	0
Subject refused[a]	6	5

[a] Some of these subjects will be seen in the near future.

[b] One of the subjects died after the assessment was completed, and one died after the social interview, but before the remaining examinations.

Table 5. Identifying Characteristics of High- and Low-Risk Subjects Participating in Full Interview

	High Risk	Low Risk
Number, full interview	173	91
Mean age at 1962 assessment	14.9	15.1
Mean social class	2.1	2.4
Number males	97	53
Number females	76	38

original sample with respect to mean age, sex distribution and social class. (see Table 2).

Deceased subjects

Of the eight deceased subjects, four are definite suicides, two suffered accidental death (disappeared from a ship, fell from a scaffold while painting a house exterior); one young woman died of an embolism. For one very recent death the cause is not yet definitely established. He was found after having been dead eight days. He was lying across his bed fully clothed. Suicide in the form of drug and alcohol poisoning is suspected. Of the eight deceased, three were in the sick group of 1967. By chance we would have expected .77 deaths from the sick group. This high mortality in the high-risk group is not in conflict with reports of frequent deaths by suicide and accidental causes among young schizophrenics (Hermansen, 1968).

Table 6. Comparison of Clinical, CAPPS and PSE Diagnoses for Subjects with High Severity of Psychopathology

Case Number	Interviewer Diagnosis	CAPPS Diagnosis	CAPPS Severity	PSE CATEGO Diagnosis	PSE CATEGO Caseness
1	Unspecified Sz. (295.9)	Schizo-affective Sz. (295.7)	5	Sz. psychosis	8
2	Hebephrenic Sz. (295.1)	Acute Sz. (295.4)	5	Sz. psychosis	8
3	Hebephrenic Sz. (295.1)	Paranoid Sz. (295.3)	6	Sz. psychosis	9
4	Hebephrenic Sz. (295.1)	Schizo-affective Sz. (295.7)	5	Sz. psychosis	9
5	Simple Sz. (295.0)	Chronic undiff. Sz. (295.9)	6	Sz. psychosis	8
6	Hebephrenic Sz. (295.1)	Paranoid Sz. (295.3)	6	Sz. psychosis	9
7	Paranoid Sz. (295.3)	Paranoid Sz. (295.3)	6	Sz. psychosis	9
8	Paranoid Sz. (295.3)	Chronic undiff. Sz. (295.9)	5	Paranoid psychosis	8
9	Schizo-affective Sz. (295.7)	Chronic undiff. Sz. (295.9)	5	Depressive psychosis	8
10	Paranoid Sz. (295.3)	Hebephrenic Sz. (295.1)	4	Sz. psychosis	8
11	Unspecified Sz. (295.9)	Acute Sz. (295.4)	4	Depressive psychosis	8
12	Paranoid Sz. (295.3)	Paranoid Sz. (295.3)	6	Depressive psychosis	9
13	Latent Sz. (295.5)	Chronic undiff. Sz. (295.9)	4	Sz. psychosis	8
14	Latent Sz. (295.5)	Chronic undiff. Sz. (295.9)	5	Paranoid psychosis	8
15	Paranoid psychosis (279.0)	Chronic undiff. Sz. (295.9)	5	Paranoid psychosis	8
16	Latent Sz. (295.5)	Chronic undiff. Sz. (295.9)	5	Paranoid psychosis	8

Note. Numbers in parentheses are World Health Organization International Classification of Disorders.

Reliability of Diagnosis

Clinical diagnosis

The interviewer's diagnostic training is basically in the classical descriptive Scandinavian classification school. A psychoanalytic personality theoretical orientation has influenced her diagnoses of the neuroses. The diagnosis of neurosis was made on the basis of positive criteria such as the presence of primary and secondary neurotic gain, circumscribed neurotic symptoms and-/or traits, and functioning defense mechanisms. The diagnosis of schizophrenia is based on the presence of Bleuler's primary symptoms: thought disorder, autism, ambivalence, and emotion blunting, as well as Bleuler's secondary symptoms: delusions and hallucinations. For a diagnosis of schizophrenia, it was not necessary that all of these symptoms were observed at the time of the interview; they might also be drawn from the anamnesis. However, thought disturbance, autism, and emotional blunting were required for a schizophrenia diagnosis. The CATEGO program classifies schizophrenia mainly on the basis of characteristic signs of delusions and hallucinations, whereas the CAPPS program places a heavy weight on any single occurence of secondary symptoms. Since the PSE only samples behavior in the month previous to the interview, and makes a conservative "diagnosis" of schizophrenia, it produced (in the high-risk group) the smallest number of schizophrenia "diagnoses", nine. The clinical diagnosis, equally conservative, but taking account of anamnestic data, diagnosed 14 schizophrenics. The CAPPS with anamnestic data and the broadest definition of schizophrenia, produced 30 schizophrenia diagnoses. The disparity between the diagnostic sources is, however, less than these figures suggest. The CAPPS has a rating of severity of illness which ranges between 1 and 6. Ratings of severity of 5 or 6 represent the most severe psychiatric illnesses. PSE has an index of "caseness" ranging from 1 to 9. Caseness indices of 8 or 9 refer to psychotic conditions. If we consider only CAPPS schizophrenia diagnoses with a severity of 5 or 6 and PSE schizophrenia "diagnoses" with a caseness of 8 or 9 and include all of the interviewer's diagnoses of schizophrenia with a caseness of 8 or 9 or a severity rating of 5 or 6 we include a total of 16 cases. These are shown in Table 6. The cases not included in this table are 2 cases clinically diagnosed as schizophrenia, but with a caseness index below 8, and some CAPPS schizophrenia diagnoses with low severity of illness ratings. Almost all of these are categorized as borderline schizophrenia*, schizoid personality disorder or paranoid personality disorder by the interviewer.

*The interviewer diagnoses borderline schizophrenia in agreement with Hoch and Polatin (1959), Knight (1954), and Vanggaard's (1958) description of the pseudoneurotic and pseudopsychopathic schizophreniform personality. The diagnosis is made in the presence of discrete thought disorder, narcissistic personal contact, pan-neurotic traits, pan-anxiety, and micropsychotic episodes.

Agreement between the clinical and CAPPS diagnosis of the subtype of schizophrenia proved to be the exception rather than the rule. However, if we consider agreement of the main diagnosis of schizophrenia (plus latent schizophrenia of high severity) there is almost a unanimity of diagnoses. There is only one of the 16 cases where disagreement occurs, case number 15. (This individual happens to be an epileptic). In this case, CAPPS diagnoses schizophrenia while the interviewer diagnoses paranoid psychosis. We conclude that agreement is excellent between the clinical interview and CAPPS for the diagnosis of schizophrenia and latent schizophrenia in severely disturbed cases.

Because it only considers pathology in the month immediately preceding the interview it is difficult to compare the PSE with the other diagnoses. Wing has developed methods for including anamnestic data in the PSE (Syndrome Check List and Aetiology Scale). When results with these scales are available, it will be possible to make direct comparisons. At this point we can indicate that all of the cases the PSE classified as schizophrenic are also diagnosed schizophrenic or latent schizophrenic by the interviewer and CAPPS. In the remaining cases it seems possible that anamnestic data would account for a part of the differences.

Since we expect between 26 or 33 schizophrenics in the high-risk group, and about half of them to have appeared in this examination, the 15 cases in Table 6 may be considered to fit our expectations.

Interrater Reliability

While we have treated the three diagnostic sources discussed immediately above as independent, they all were the product of the interviewer's coding and judgment. Consequently we have planned work on interrater reliability. We can report early results of this work. A psychiatrist, Raben Rosenberg, listened to the audio tape of the 3 ¼-hour interview, read the case material and made a diagnosis of ten randomly selected cases. The primary and secondary diagnoses for the interviewer and Dr. Rosenberg are presented in Table 7. Agreement between the diagnoses is rather good especially in the light of the range of diagnoses present.

Fate of Sick, Well, and Control Groups

The sick group consisted of a variety of psychiatric conditions: schizophrenia, odd personalities, delinquent, and alcoholic boys. The well and control group consisted of high- and low-risk subjects who were showing good adjustment at the time of the 1967 followup.

The WHO (1967) diagnostic system has no class for borderline schizophrenia, which has to be assigned to the latent schizophrenias 295.59.

Table 7.   Comparison of Independent Diagnoses Made by Interviewer and Second Diagnostician on Ten Cases

Subject	Dr. Rosenberg's Diagnosis	Interviewer's Diagnosis
H 1	No mental disorder Alt.: Characterneurosis obs. pro.	Personality disorder unspecified obs. pro. Alt.: No mental disorder
L 2	Characterneurosis	Obsessive compulsive characterneurosis
H 3	Paranoid personality disorder Alt.: Latent schizophrenia obs. pro.	Paranoid personality disorder Alt.: Latent schizophrenia
L 4	No mental disorder Alt.: Hysterical neurosis	No mental disorder Alt.: Hysterical neurosis
H 5	Depressive neurosis Alt.: Affective personality disorder	Paranoid personality disorder
H 6	Depressive neurosis Alt.: Characterneurosis	Personality disorder, unspecified Alt.: Schizoid personality disorder obs. pro.
L 7	Schizoid personality disorder Alt.: Characterneurosis obs. pro.	Characterneurosis Alt.: No mental illness
H 8	Latent schizophrenia Alt.: Schizoid personality disorder	Schizoid personality disorder Alt.: Latent schizophrenia
L 9	No mental illness Alt.: Obsessive compulsive character-neurosis obs. pro.	No mental illness Alt.: Obsessive compulsive character-neurosis obs. pro.
H 10	Hebephrenic schizophrenia Alt.: Paranoid schizophrenia	Paranoid schizophrenia

The interviewer (blind to the group identification of these subjects) diagnosed 6 of the 20 in the sick group as schizophrenic, 6 as latent schizophrenic, 1 as paranoia, 6 as personality disorders and 1 as hysterical neurosis. Three of the 20 have committed suicide; all of the suicides were diagnosed schizophrenic, one on the basis of this interview, two on the basis of other evidence.

In the well group none have died. The interviewer diagnosed 2 of the 20 as schizophrenic, 3 as latent schizophrenic, 4 as personality disorder, 5 as neurotic, and 4 as having no mental illness. One of the well subjects refused to be interviewed and another was abroad at the time this paper was written.

None of the controls were diagnosed by the interviewer as schizophrenic or as latent schizophrenic. Five were diagnosed as having personality disorders,

11 as neurotic, and 3 as having no mental illness. One refused to participate in the assessment. A detailed statement on the fate of the sick, well and control groups is being prepared for separate publication.

Distinguishing Premorbid Characteristics of the Schizophrenics

The followup has identified schizophrenia among the 207 high-risk subjects. As the time of this writing we have three sources of diagnoses of schizophrenia; they show good agreement at least for the serious cases. For purposes of this paper we determined to make a preliminary analysis of the premorbid characteristics of the schizophrenics. In as much as the interviewer's diagnosis of schizophrenia overlapped most with the other diagnostic sources and proved to be the most moderate diagnostic source we utilized the interviewer's diagnoses for purposes of this preliminary analysis. In future publications we intend to compare analyses using the various diagnostic sources.

In the high-risk group the interviewer diagnosed 14 schizophrenics. (Twelve of these 14 are among the 15 agreed upon as schizophrenic by at least two diagnostic sources). These 14 schizophrenics were compared with the interviewer's 29 borderline schizophrenics, 34 neurotics, and 23 with no mental illness. For purposes of this analysis only the high-risk group was considered. The data analyzed consisted of information concerning factors relating to the schizophrenic mother's hospitalization, the pregnancy and delivery of the subject, the early childhood, family relations, and teacher's judgment of the subject.

We should emphasize both the tentativeness of this report and the fact that the findings may relate more to "early onset" than to "late onset" schizophrenia. We should also again point out that these analyses refer only to the interviewer's diagnoses.

The 14 high-risk subjects who were diagnosed schizophrenic (schizophrenic group) had mothers whose illness began while the mother was relatively young. She was also younger at the time of her first hospitalization. This suggests that the mothers of the schizophrenic group had a more chronic and serious illness. As we have stated earlier this finding lends itself to both genetic and environmental interpretations (Mednick & Schulsinger, 1968).

The birth of the schizophrenic group was relatively difficult. The period of labor was longer and was characterized by more complications. It should also be mentioned that the mothers of the schizophrenics were more frequently unmarried.

The rearing social class of the schizophrenic group was not noticeably different from that of the other three groups. No significant differences were observed on individual items relating to early infant behavior or parental attitudes or behavior. It was noticed that the schizophrenic group did evidence marginally greater deviance on a number of items reflecting infant behavior.

However, not one of these differences was statistically significant. It is possible that a scale combining these deviant items will prove of interest. It should be pointed out that of the 14 schizophrenics only 2 had been raised in an intact family.

Except for the perinatal data (based on midwife reports), all of the results above are based on retrospective reports. As such they must be accepted with caution. The school teacher who rated the behavior of the subjects, however, based his or her report on the current behavior of the subject (true for approximately 50% of the sample) or on the basis of relatively short-term retrospection, backed up by the school records and the fact that in most cases the teachers had known the subjects for a period of years.

On the whole the schizophrenic group separated itself sharply from the other groups in the teachers' judgments. They were reported as being very easily angered and upset and very slow in calming down from such upsets. The schizophrenic group disturbed the class with inappropriate behavior, was characterized as being violent and aggressive and a disciplinary problem for the teacher. The teacher was asked to predict whether the pupil would suffer a serious mental illness in the future. The teacher made this judgment in the case of 6% of the no mental illness and neurotic groups, 21% of the borderline group, and 33% of the schizophrenic group.

Implications

As is indicated in the introduction to this chapter, the high-risk studies have as their most important function their contribution to research on prevention. They contribute in two ways: (1) identification of premorbid signs, which may make possible the early detection, in the general population, of individuals at very high risk for schizophrenia, (2) by consideration of these premorbid signs the method can suggest modes of interventive activity.

This function of high-risk studies is well illustrated by an intervention project currently being attempted. A group of investigators (Mednick, Raman, Schulsinger, Sutton-Smith, Venables, & Bell) is investigating prevention methods with high-risk children on the island of Mauritius (Bell, et al., 1975; Schulsinger, et al., in press). The purpose of the project is to select from the results of a population survey, 3-year-old children at high risk for psychological disorder, place these high-risk children into therapeutic nursery schools, engage in specific controlled intervention, and follow these children to observe their long-term outcome. Because of the age of the children and the probable cross-cultural stability of the measures, we used psychophysiological techniques to pick our high-risk children. We chose three-year-old children whose psychophysiological deviance was similar to that of the subjects of the Copenhagen project who had suffered psychiatric breakdown. It was our assumption that a Mauritian sample of three-year-olds who exhibit such autonomic deviance would also be at risk for breakdown. The investigators are not totally blind to the weaknesses of this assumption. However, the longitudinal study of three year olds whose autonomic characteristics have been recorded was deemed a worthy effort in its own right.

Description of Mauritius

Mauritius is a densely populated country with about 900,000 inhabitants occupying an area of approximately 2400 square kilometers and is located some 1000 kilometers east of Madagascar on latitude 20° south. The population is composed of Hindus and Tamils (51%), Moslems (16%), Creoles (29%), and Chinese (4%). The economy is at present not advanced and is largely dependent on the cultivation of sugar cane. The annual per capita income is about US $220. In spite of this the infrastructure is quite advanced. Perinatal care is of a relatively high standard. Some 90% of the children attend elementary school for several years. Emigration is limited. Infections and parasitic disorders are relatively well under control. Mild malnutrition (hypoproteinemia) is common, but pronounced kwashiorkor or marasmus is rare.

There is approximately one psychiatric hospital bed per 1000 inhabitants, a ratio far higher than in other developing countries. The climate is subtropical to tropical. Foreigners manage well with French or English, since both are official languages. The indigenous population speaks a variety of patois. In some rural areas Hindi is the major language.

Description of Assessment

From August, 1972 through July, 1973 we examined 1800 three-year-old children from two neighboring Mauritian municipalities, Quatre Bornes and Vacoas. These 1800 children comprise almost the complete population of three-year-old children in these municipalities. The testing program for each child consisted of a number of laboratory tests and the collection of social and medical information. The various examinations are summarized below:

1.   *The Parent Interview.*   This was a field interview with the parent on which judgments were made concerning the health and living conditions of the family. In all there were 55 items, which covered the occupational status of the parents, their educational history, and the living accomodation of the family. The interview also included items about siblingship, etc.

2.   *Social Behavior Observation.*   This procedure was carried out while the child was in the playroom and waiting room. It consisted of a checklist of items that covered the relationship between the child and his parent and other children. The extent to which the child used the various toys was also noted.

3. *Psychological Assessment.*   This was a modified procedure from that which had been developed for use with Puerto Rican children in New York. It included tests of manipulation, color naming, and conservation. The test was carried out in the local patois and, on occasion, in Hindi. The parent was present during the test.

4. *Psychophysiology Test.*   Each child who was examined at the laboratory provided a physiological record obtained from a standard orienting and conditioning paradigm. The child listened to a series of tones presented over stereo headphones. The stimulus tape comprised 6 orienting and 18 conditioning trials. The physiological parameters (which included skin conductance (SC), skin potential (SP), and the electrocardiogram (EKG)) were monitored continuously during presentation of the tape, which lasted approximately 20 minutes.

5. *Electroencephalography Examination.*   Two occipital leads were monitored under resting conditions for approximately 10 minutes for each child. (The EEG work was supervised by George Ulett and Turan Itil.)

6. *The Laboratory Behavior Questionnaire.*   This was largely intended as a checklist in which the ambient temperature and humidity of the laboratory together with other technical details concerning apparatus performance could be noted. Additionally, we included items covering the child's reaction to the testing (whether he cried or was agitated, the extent to which tremor was evident in the limbs). Methodological points dealing with electrode placement and function were also made on this form.

7. *The Obstetric Information Questionnaire.*   The items on this questionnaire were completed from ante-natal and delivery cards maintained by the local health authorities. Information was available for 60% of the entire sample. Items included information about the pregnancy and the delivery (e.g., the occurrence of anemia and albuminuria, the fetal presentation, and weight at birth).

8. *Pediatric Examination.*   The examination was carried out by a group of Mauritian doctors. Our interest was essentially to obtain information that related to the nutritional status of the child. Particular emphasis was therefore given to items concerning malnutrition and the presence of worm infestations. We used as indicators of these states those symptoms commonly noted in a tropical environment: for example, whether facial edema was present, skin folds, angular stomatitis, and the condition and pigmentation status of the hair.* Laboratory determination of blood and urine samples provided informa-

*The reddish hair color often associated with malnutrition is recognized in Mauritian folklore as a sign of religious significance: it is commonly referred to as "cheveux de Bon Dieu".

tion of hemoglobin values and the occurrence of sugar and albumin.

The data amount to approximately 130,000 IBM cards, and it will take some time before they are analyzed. First of all, we had to select the children for our experimental preventive intervention.

From each of the two municipalities we selected 100 children. Of these 56 showed abnormally fast psychophysiological recovery, 12 were psychophysiological nonresponders, and the remaining 32 were psychophysiologically normals or "low risk." In each of the two municipalities we have established a well-equipped nursery school.† Each nursery school caters for 50 of the 100 selected children in each of the municipalities and the remaining 50 will serve as controls. During the first year in nursery school systematic observations are made of the childrens' behavior in a variety of situations, in order to establish a base line.

On the basis of this we intend, during the last year before these children enter primary school, to expose them to a variety of interventions. One of these will be a program of behavior training. Another will consist of systematic compensations for social disruptions in the home environment. We also consider the possibility of having younger playmates for some of the risk children. Preventive use of neuroleptic drugs has been considered, but also rejected. No neuroleptic drug without undesirable side effects is known today. Neither do we know what children could be deprived of under long-lasting neuroleptic influence.

It will be possible to follow the 100 nursery school and the 100 non nursery school children into their adult life, and to correlate variations in outcome to differences in their childhood experience and subsequent life conditions. Our impression at the moment (i.e., during the behavior observation phase) is that the nursery school where sufficient education and food is provided is in itself a very powerful and beneficial intervention. In addition to the preventive program, a project that surveys the physical, mental, and social conditions of 1800 three-year-old children in a developing country with a built-in opportunity to follow them all has its own value.

REFERENCES

Atkinson, R. L. & Robinson, N. M. Paired-associate learning by schizophrenic and normal subjects under conditions of personal and impersonal reward and punishment. *Journal of Abnormal and Social Psychology,* 1961, **62,** 322–326.

Ax, A. F. & Bamford, J. L. The GSR recovery limb in chronic schizophrenics. *Psychophysiology,* 1970, **7,** 145–147.

†The nursery schools are supported by the Danish Government as a development project. The Danish pedagogical experts train the first 14 Mauritian nursery school teachers.

Bader-Bartfai, A. & Schalling, D. Recovery times of skin conductance responses as related to some personality and physiological variables. Psychological Institute, University of Stockholm, 1974.

Bagshaw, M. H. & Kimble, D. Bimodal EDR orienting response characteristics of limbic lesioned monkeys: correlates with schizophrenic patients. Paper presented at the Annual Meeting of the Society for Psychophysiological Research, 1972.

Bell, B., Mednick, S., Raman, A. C., Schulsinger, F., Sutton-Smith, B., & Venables, P. A longitudinal psychophysiological study of three year-old Mauritian children: Preliminary report. *Developmental Medicine and Child Neurology,* 1975, **17**, 320–324.

Cavanaugh, D. K. Improvement in the performance of schizophrenics on concept formation tasks as a function of motivational change. *Journal of Abnormal and Social Psychology,* 1958, **57**, 8–12.

Crain, A. J., Sussmann, M. B., & Weil, W. B., Jr. Effects of a diabetic child on marital integration and related measures of family functioning. *Journal of Health and Human Behavior,* 1966a, **67**, 122–127.

Crain, A. J., Sussmann, M. B. & Weil, W. B., Jr. Family interaction, diabetes and sibling relationship. *International Journal of Social Psychiatry,* 1966b, **12**, 35–43.

Darrow, C. W. The equation of the galvanic skin reflex curve: I. The dynamics of reaction in relation to excitation-background. *Journal of General Psychology,* 1937, **16**, 285.

Endicott, J. & Spitzer, R. Current and Past Psychopathology Scales (CAPPS), *Achives of General Psychiatry,* **27**, Nov. 1972.

Fontana, A. F. Familial etiology of schizophrenia: Is a scientific methodology possible? *Psychological Bulletin,* 1966, 64, 214–227.

Freeman, G. L. and Katzoff, E. T. Methodological evalution of the GSR with special reference to the formula for R.Q. (recovery quotient). *Journal of Experimental Psychology,* 1942, **31**, 239–248.

Furedy, J. J. Electrodermal recovery time as a supra-sensitive autonomic index of anticipated intensity of threatened shock. *Psychophysiology,* 1972, **9**, 281–282.

Goldfarb, C. & Erlenmeyer-Kimling, L. Changing mating and fertility patterns in schizophrenia. in F.J. Kallman (Ed.) *Expanding goals of genetics in psychiatry.* New York: Grune and Stratton, 1962.

Gruzelier, J. H. Bilateral asymmetry of skin conductance orienting activity and levels in schizophrenics. *Biological Psychology,* 1973a, **1**, 21–42.

Gruzelier, J. H. The investigation of possible limbic dysfunction in schizophrenia by psychophysiological methods. Unpublished Ph.D. thesis, University of London, 1973b.

Gruzelier, J. H. & Venables, P. H. Skin conductance orienting activity in a heterogeneous sample of schizophrenics. Possible evidence of limbic dysfunction. *Journal of Nervous and Mental Disease,* 1972, **155**, 277–287.

Hare, R. D. Personal communication, 1974.

Hermansen, L. Suicides among schizophrenics. *Nordisk Psykiatrisk Tidsskrift,* 1968, **XXII,** 4, 324–337.

Heston, L. L. Psychiatric disorders in foster home reared children of schizophrenic mothers. *British Journal of Psychiatry,* 1966, **112,** 819–825.

Higgins, J. Effect of child rearing by schizophrenic mothers. *Journal of Psychiatric Research,* 1966, **4,** 153–167.

Hoch, P. H. & Palatin, Z. P. Pseudoneurotic forms of schizophrenia. *Psychiatric Quarterly,* 1949, **23,** 248–276.

Janes, C. L. & Stern, J. A. Electrodermal response configuration as a function of rated psychopathology in children. (In press.)

Johannesen, W. J. Motivation in schizophrenic performance: A review. *Psychological Reports,* 1964, **15,** 839–870.

Kallmann, F. J. *The genetics of schizophrenia.* New York: Augustin, 1938.

Kallmann, F. J. The genetic theory of schizophrenia. *American Journal of Psychiatry,* 1946, **103,** 309–322.

Kammerer, P. C. An exploratory study of crippled children. *Psychological Record,* 1940, **4,** 47–100.

Kessler, P. & Neale, J. M. Hippocampal damage and schizophrenia: A critique of Mednick's theory. *Journal of Abnormal Psychology,* 1974, **83,** 91–96.

Kirkegaard-Sorensen, L. & Mednick, S. A. Registered criminality in families of children at high risk for schizophrenia. *Journal of Abnormal Psychology,* in press.

Knight, R. P. Borderling States. In R. P. Knight and C. R. Friedman (Eds.), *Psychoanalytic psychiatry and psychology.* New York: International University Press, 1954.

Lewis, A. J. The offspring of parents both mentally ill. *Acta Geneticae,* 1959, **7,** 309–322.

Losen, S. M. The differential effects of censure on the problem solving behavior of schizophrenic and normal subjects. *Journal of Personality,* 1961, **29,** 258–272.

Mattson, A. & Gross, S. Adaptional and defensive behavior in young hemophiliacs and their parents. *American Journal of Psychiatry,* 1966, **122,** 1349–1356.

McLardy, T. Deficit and paucity of dentate granule-cells in some schizophrenic brains. *International Research Communication System,* March, 1973.

Mednick, S. A. A learning theory approach to research in schizophrenia. *Psychological Bulletin,* 1958, **55,** 316–327.

Mednick, S. A. Schizophrenia: A learned thought disorder. In G. S. Nielsen (Ed.), *Clinical psychology, Proceedings of the XIV international congress of applied psychology. Vol. 4. Clinical Psychology.* Copenhagen: Munksgaard, 1962.

Mednick, S. A. Breakdown in individuals at high risk for schizophrenia: Possible predispositional perinatal factors. *Mental Hygiene,* 1970, **54,** 50–63.

Mednick, S. A. Electrodermal recovery and psychopathology. In S. A. Mednick et al. (Eds.), *Genetics, environment, and psychopathology.* Amsterdam: North Holland, 1974.

Mednick, S. A. & Loeb, J. Unpublished manuscript.

Mednick, S. A. & McNeil, T. F. Current methodology in research on the etiology of schizophrenia: Serious difficulties which suggest the use of the high-risk group method. *Psychological Bulletin,* 1968, **70,** 681–693.

Mednick, S. A., Mura, E., Schulsinger, F., & Mednick, B. Perinatal conditions and infant development in children with schizophrenic parents. *Social Biology,* 1971, **18,** 103–113.

Mednick, S. A. & Schulsinger, F. Children of schizophrenic mothers. *Bulletin of the International Association of Applied Psychology,* 1965a, **14,** 11–27.

Mednick, S. A. & Schulsinger, F. A longitudinal study of children with a high risk for schizophrenia: A preliminary report. In S. Vandenberg (Ed.), *Methods and goals in human behavior genetics.* New York: Academic Press, 1965b, pp. 255–296.

Mednick, S. A. & Schulsinger, F. Some premorbid characteristics related to breakdown in children with schizophrenic mothers. *Journal of Psychiatric Research,* 1968, **6,** (Suppl. 1), 267–291.

Mednick, S. A., Schulsinger, F., Higgins, J., & Bell, B. *Genetics, environment, and psychopathology.* Amsterdam: North Holland/ American Elsevier, 1974.

Murphy, H. B. M. & Raman, A. C. The chronicity of schizophrenia in indigenous tropical peoples. Results of a twelve-year follow-up survey. *British Journal of Psychiatry,* 1971, **118,** 489–98.

Novelly, R. A., Graham, J. J., & Ax, A. F. Psychophysiological correlates of temporal lobe epilepsy. Paper presented to the Psychophysiological Society Meeting. Salt Lake City, 1974.

Reisby, N. Psychoses in children of schizophrenic mothers. *Acta Psychiatrica Scandinavica,* 1967, **43,** 8–20.

Rodnick, E. & Garmezy, N. An experimental approach to the study of motivation in schizophrenia. In M. R. Jones (Ed.), *Nebraska Symposium on Motivation.* Lincoln: University of Nebraska Press, 1957.

Rosenbaum, S. Z. Infantile paralysis as a source of emotional problems in children. *Welfare Bulletin,* 1943, **34,** 11–13.

Schalling, D. & Levander, S. Spontaneous fluctuations in skin conductance during anticipation of pain in two delinquent groups, differing in anxiety-proneness. Reports from Psychological Laboratories, the University of Stockholm 1967, No. 238.

Schulsinger, F. et al. The early detection and prevention of mental illness: The Mauritius Project. A preliminary report. *Neuropsychobiology.* In press.

Schulz, B. Empirische Untersuchungen über die beidseitigen Belastung mit endogenen Psychosen. *Zeitschrift für Neurologie und Psychiatie,* 1939, **165,** 97–108.

Schulz, B. Kinder schizophrener Elternpaare. *Zeitschrift für Neurologie und Psychiatrie,* 1940, **168,** 332–381.

Spain, B. Eyelid conditioning and arousal in schizophrenic and normal subjects. *Journal of Abnormal Psychology,* 1966, **71,** 260–266.

Svalastoga, K. *Prestige, class and mobility.* Copenhagen: Gyldendal, 1959.

Vanggaard, T. Neurosis and Pseudoneurosis. *Acta Psychiatrica et Neurologica Scandinavica,* 1958, **33,** 251–254.

Venables, P. H. In S. A. Mednick et al. (Eds.), *Genetics, environment, and psychopathology.* Amsterdam: North Holland, 1974.

Wing, J. K., Cooper, J. E., & Sartorius, N. The measurement and classification of psychiatric symptoms. New York: Cambridge University Press, 1974.

World Health Organization. *Manual of the International Statistical Classification of Diseases, Injuries, and Causes of Death, Vol. 1,* Eighth Revision, Geneva: World Health Organization, 1967.

Yolles, S. & Kramer, M. Vital Statistics. In L. Bellak and L. Loeb (Eds.): *The schizophrenic syndrome,* New York: Grune and Stratton, 1969.

Index